Quality of Life

Occupational Therapy in Chronic Condition Management, Palliative Care, and Hospice

Edited by **Lindsey Buddelmeyer, OTD, MOT, OTR/L**

American Occupational Therapy Association

AOTA Vision 2025
As an inclusive profession, occupational therapy maximizes health, well-being, and quality of life for all people, populations, and communities through effective solutions that facilitate participation in everyday living.

Mission Statement
The American Occupational Therapy Association advances occupational therapy practice, education, and research through standard-setting and advocacy on behalf of its members, the profession, and the public.

AOTA Staff
Sherry Keramidas, *Executive Director*
Matthew Clark, *Chief Officer, Innovation & Engagement*

Elizabeth Dooley, *Vice President, Strategic Marketing & Communications*
Laura Collins, *Director of Communications and Publications*
Ashley Hofmann, *Acquisitions & Development Manager, AOTA Press*
Amy Ricci, *Product Manager & Business Analyst, AOTA Press*

Rebecca Rutberg, *Director, Marketing*
Amanda Goldman, *Marketing Manager*
Jennifer Folden, *Brand Designer*

American Occupational Therapy Association, Inc.
6116 Executive Boulevard, Suite 200
North Bethesda, MD 20852-4929
www.aota.org
To order: 1-800-729-AOTA (2682) or store.aota.org

ISBN: 978-1-56900-628-3
eBOOK ISBN: 978-1-56900-629-0
Library of Congress Control Number: 2023932720

Cover design by Steve Parrish, AOTA, North Bethesda, MD
Composition by Manila Typesetting Company, Manila, Philippines
Printed and bound by CPI Group (UK) Ltd, Croydon, CR0 4YY

Suggested citation: Buddelmeyer, L. (Ed.). (2023). *Quality of life: Occupational therapy in chronic condition management, palliative care, and hospice.* AOTA Press.

Dedication

To my husband—when I asked you 2 years ago about the idea of writing a book about chronic illness and palliative care, you looked at me without hesitation and said, "Why wouldn't you?" You believe in me more than I believe in myself and always see the best in me. I will love you forever.

To my four beautiful children, Alexis, Ava, James, and Zechariah—you give me inspiration every day, and I adore you. You are my greatest blessings in life, and I couldn't love you more.

Lastly, this book is dedicated to all patients and families who have or are facing chronic illness. It is a hard-fought battle that by no means goes unnoticed. We see you . . . we hear you . . . and we acknowledge that there are opportunities for us to do better, so that we may serve any and ALL individuals facing a life-long illness.

Contents

Acknowledgements

To my parents, Steve and Christine—thank you for your love, support, and strength. Your selfless acts of caregiving and doing for others has helped guide me on my path to serving others. I love you further than the moon.

To my mother-in-law, Marvelle, and late father-in-law, Jimmy—I have watched your battle with chronic illness as caregiver and patient. I love you both. Jimmy, you were also an inspiration for this book, we sure do miss you.

To my amazing team of authors, I am forever grateful for you sharing your many talents with the hopes that a body of work such as this will perhaps one day serve as a guide and resource for those facing and working with chronic illness.

I would like to acknowledge my incredible editor, Ashley Hofmann, the Acquisitions & Development Manager for AOTA Press. You have understood the vision for this book from day one. You have been an amazing force to help guide me through this process. I am so grateful to have had the opportunity to work with you.

List of Figures, Tables, Exhibits, and Case Examples

FIGURES

TABLES

EXHIBITS

CASE EXAMPLES

About the Editor

Lindsey Buddelmeyer, OTD, MOT, OTR/L, is the Leadership Education & Training Specialist at Blanchard Valley Health System (BVHS) in Findlay, Ohio. She has a personal and professional passion for advocating and working with the chronic disease community. Previously, she has worked as a full-time faculty member at the University of Findlay, and as an adjunct for St. Catherine University in its postprofessional doctorate program. Lindsey also worked as an occupational therapist on the palliative care team for 4 years at Bridge Palliative Care and Hospice. Lindsey has been certified in the caregiver education and training program, Skills2Care, and successfully embedded this program and occupational therapy services into palliative care practice through a grant that she received from the Hancock County Community Foundation in Findlay.

Lindsey is also trained as a Dementia Friend and provides the Dementia Friends education and training for the lay and professional communities. Lindsey is strategically working to train volunteers and nurses at BVHS to become Dementia Friends. This work also ties into a project that she has been a part of in conjunction with the University of Findlay's Mazza Museum in which hospital volunteers are trained as Dementia Friends and then take children's literature books from the Mazza Museum out to skilled nursing, assisted living, and memory care units of the health system to read books with residents and create paintings based off them or long-term memory retrieval and experiences. There is a dedicated space in the Mazza Museum called the *1-2-3 Remember Me Wall* in which these works of art are showcased.

Lindsey has served as a consultant and continues her work with the Ohio Council for Cognitive Health. Lindsey has been published and presented at both the state and national levels during the past 10 years of her career. These experiences and platforms have included a wide range of community and professional organizations involving topics surrounding chronic illness, palliative care, and hospice. Most notably she has presented at the Annual Assembly for Hospice and Palliative Care, the American Occupational Therapy Association's Annual Conference & Expo, and has provided continuing medical education for physicians on the role of occupational therapy practitioners in palliative care practice.

Introduction

LINDSEY BUDDELMEYER, OTD, MOT, OTR/L

Chronic diseases in America are the leading causes of death and disability and are responsible for driving annual health care costs to $4.1 trillion dollars (Centers for Disease Control and Prevention [CDC], 2022). An alarming 6 in 10 adults are living with a chronic illness (CDC, 2022). By its very design, the traditional medical model is set up to be more reactive than proactive, which lends itself to an abundance of shortcomings related to best practices and the chronic disease community. In addition, updated policies and practices, such as the Quadruple Aim and value-based care, are forcing health care stakeholders to examine and evaluate the inner-workings of the quality of care that they offer and provide. An integral part of this reexamination process should involve the evolution and expansion of more contemporized models of health care, such as considering a different protocol, model, and practice in dealing with high-risk populations. Skilled care involving occupational therapy services should be a standard part of palliative care and hospice care versus only ordering and using such services with a rehabilitative mindset.

How This Book Emerged

I waited in a line that wrapped around the church and out the door to say my final good-byes. This line gave me time to stand and reflect on my experiences with Sandy. This one hurt. Sandy was a patient of mine that I had worked with for approximately 5 years under a community-based palliative care practice model. I had gotten to know Sandy and her family well. Her beautiful family was her most prized possession, and they all stood in a line together, united to say their good-byes.

As I watched the images of Sandy flash before me on several flat screen TVs, I had a lump in my throat and tears in my eyes. I finally came face-to-face with Sandy's daughter, Jodi. When she saw me, she said, "You were there, there in the beginning. You helped us face so many uncertainties and obstacles along the way. As I think back, I can't imagine a time that you weren't there for my mother or my family. Thank you for all that you did for her and for us. She fought so hard, and she loved you so much." The tears got larger as they ricocheted down my cheeks; the gravity of her loss and all that we had done together felt incredibly heavy.

With Sandy and her family, I had witnessed the highs and lows that accompany chronic illness. This was yet another example of a case that I had entered in which the patient and family were in a state of crisis. As an occupational therapist, I am too often called in to do an evaluation at the point at which things have already snowballed out of control, with unmanaged symptoms, compromised quality of life (QoL), poor medication management, risk for falls, and caregivers grappling with a role for which they have no formal training or support. In these situations, it is not a matter of if hospitalization will occur, but rather when hospitalization will occur. But for Sandy, it was different. In the beginning to the middle stages of Sandy's illness, she could engage in meaningful conversations related to advance directives and care planning. These conversations would unknowingly help guide the incredibly difficult decisions that were ahead. During a palliative care session, Sandy was very clear that if it came to a point in her illness that she was no longer eating, she did not want a feeding tube. In the advanced stages of her illness, this is the space in which Sandy and her family found themselves; she simply wasn't eating. Although the pain of the decision to forego a feeding tube was very hard, Sandy's wishes were clear, and there was no confusion. In the end, Sandy's wishes were honored.

I realized that I journeyed alongside Sandy and her family from the beginning to the end of her chronic illness, working to facilitate QoL all along the way. This is how I envision all chronic care to be. Sandy was able to receive palliative care services from the time that she began to experience symptoms through end-of-life care, at which point she transitioned to hospice. She had a team of experts (physician, nurse practitioner, social worker, spiritual care, occupational therapist) in her corner along a continuum of care. Skilled care as a key player in a maintenance type of approach was uncharted territory. My role as an occupational therapist had been to advocate, educate, guide, empower, adapt and grade functional tasks, and provide caregiver education and training—all to maintain and preserve QoL for both Sandy and her caregivers. The ultimate goal was to keep everyone supported, so Sandy could remain in her home and out of the hospital for as long as possible. Palliative care and hospice provide the platform for me to serve and support patients along the continuum of care.

Sandy will always be one of my most treasured cases for so many reasons, many of which you will come to know and understand as you dig more into the pages of this book and get to know more about Sandy as well as others who have so bravely fought with chronic illness or fought for someone living with chronic illness. Far too often, the wishes of our patients are sacrificed, and QoL becomes overlooked. More contemporized models of care better positions patients' wishes to be heard and empowers them to play an active role in the management of their health.

Terminology

In this text, the term *occupational therapy practitioner* encompasses both occupational therapists and occupational therapy assistants. In addition, the editor made a conscious choice to use the term *patient* instead of *client* throughout the text because this is a more universally understood term in the health care arena among a wide range of health care professionals. It is hoped that this book will serve as a resource beyond the occupational therapy community!

How This Book Is Organized

The book begins with an overview of health care reform and policy in Chapter 1, "Improving Outcomes: Health Care Reform and Occupational Therapy in Palliative Care and Hospice." This is followed by a detailed look into the chronic disease community and the importance that occupational therapy practitioners place on building therapeutic relationships. An overarching view about palliative care and hospice follow to give the reader an understanding of the evolution and current practice of these models of care. The application of occupational therapy services under palliative care and then hospice are covered in detail. These readings involve eligibility, referral, application, and more to help readers conceptualize what occupational therapy practice looks like under palliative care and hospice. Lastly, Chapter 7, "Caregivers and Occupational Therapy: A

Vital Partnership," examines the incredibly important role of the caregiver and describes how we can employ best practice to help, support, and guide this interdependent role between patient and caregiver.

A Vision for the Future

> *If there's a book that you want to read, but it hasn't been written yet, then you must write it.* —Toni Morrison

Occupational therapy practitioners have a distinct role on teams in chronic condition management, palliative care, and hospice to identify and assess functional decline and challenges to help further support the mission and practice of chronic disease models of care. By better understanding these spaces, it is hoped that more occupational therapy practitioners will not only be proactive and step up but also be invited to the table.

These pages hold the spirit and passion of health care professionals who wholeheartedly believe that, beyond the traditional medical model, there is a better way to serve patients facing chronic illness. This text serves as a foundation to better understanding the policy, practice, and inner-workings of chronic illness, palliative care, and hospice. We have much work to do.

REFERENCE

Centers for Disease Control and Prevention. (2022). *Chronic diseases in America.* https://www.cdc.gov/chronicdisease/pdf/infographics/chronic-disease-in-america-H.pdf

1

Improving Outcomes: Health Care Reform and Occupational Therapy in Palliative Care and Hospice

AMY J. LAMB, OTD, OTR/L, FAOTA

Learning Objectives

After completing this chapter, readers will be able to

- understand how improving outcomes can reduce cost,
- describe the Triple Aim and how palliative care and hospice contribute to the Triple Aim,
- define the Quadruple Aim,
- explain the role of advanced care planning, and
- advocate for including occupational therapy in the Palliative Care and Hospice Education and Training Act.

Key Terms and Concepts

advanced care planning
Center to Advance Palliative Care
compassion fatigue
hospice care
Mobile Integrated Healthcare Community Paramedicine program
palliative care
Palliative Care and Hospice Education and Training Act
palliative care teams
Patient Protection and Affordable Care Act
Quadruple Aim
quality of life
Triple Aim

The 2010 ***Patient Protection and Affordable Care Act*** (ACA; P. L. 111-148) has altered the policy and practice landscape since its passage and implementation, including the practice of occupational therapy and the role of palliative care and hospice in meeting the needs of patients served as part of occupational therapy practice. Occupational therapy professionals are required to understand the role that palliative care and hospice play and how the strategies of these often underused parts of the health care system can be better used to promote quality of life (QoL) for patients with serious chronic illness or terminal diagnoses and their families.

There are an estimated 45 million Americans diagnosed with one or more chronic conditions that are likely to not only get progressively worse over time but that also limit personal function (Institute of Medicine [IOM], 2015; National Academies of Sciences, Engineering, and Medicine, 2016). As a result, QoL is often negatively affected. The World Health Organization (WHO; 2023) defines ***QoL*** as "an individual's perception of their position in life in the context of the culture and value systems in which they live and in relation to their goals, expectations, standards and concerns." The U.S. health care delivery system continues to focus primarily on treating acute and curable conditions, compared to supporting daily functioning and QoL (Cohn et al., 2017). However, palliative and hospice care share common ground in their focus on preserving QoL for patients and caregivers. ***Palliative care*** is a specialized area of medicine designed for people living with chronic illness. Relief from symptoms and stress associated with the illness are its key features (Center to Advance Palliative Care, 2023). ***Hospice care*** can be provided along the continuum of palliative care; it is geared more toward end of life once it has been determined that the illness is terminal and the patient wishes to forgo curative treatment (Center for Improving Value in Health Care, 2012).

The U.S. health care system has long been focused on curative care, and it is often not well integrated with palliative and hospice care delivery models. Many health care providers lack exposure to and understanding of palliative care in the management of serious and chronic illness or of hospice in the management of terminal illness. This lack leaves a knowledge gap between providers and the front-line health care workforce supporting individuals in understanding the options available to them on the continuum of care and having conversations with patients about preferences for care and end-of-life planning.

Viewed through the reimbursement lens, the value-based payment models that have grown out of health care reform in recent years have provided a new opportunity to integrate palliative care into health care systems. Heo et al. (2022) documented how value-based care opened the door for palliative care providers to receive more inclusive reimbursement. Historically, the Medicare Hospice Benefit was a primary access point and payer. However, value-based payment creates a bridge for payers to now pay for palliative care, which fills an important gap in the health care continuum.

This chapter explores the role of the Triple Aim in the foundation of the ACA and how it can serve as a bridge for providers and payers in palliative and hospice care, focusing on how palliative care and hospice improve the patient experience, contribute to health, and reduce health care costs.

Improving Outcomes to Reduce Cost

Advances in modern medicine have altered how patients experience chronic illness and end-of-life care. Although these medical advances have lengthened the length of time people may live, the QoL of both patients and their loved ones has frequently been questioned. The increasing complexity of medical challenges and their impact on patients have added to the epidemic of caregiver burden (Warraich et al., 2017).

Previous data have shown that approximately one-quarter of Medicare spending in the United States occurs in the last year of a person's life. End-of-life spending is complex and costly. Although a person with a chronic disease might spend an average of $57,000 per year on their health care, a person with cancer undergoing treatment may spend up to $25,000 in the first month (Joynt et al., 2017). Spending money on intensive health care for sick people can save the lives of many, and it is fundamentally a good thing and part of the reason the health care system exists. With that said, an important conversation for patients and families concerns the best decision for them given the available tools, resources, and information. Palliative care has been shown to increase patients' satisfaction with the care they receive, and it is linked to medical expense cost savings and reduced need for hospitalization, rehabilitation, and trips to the emergency department (Hughes & Smith, 2014).

The benefits of palliative care can include improvement in QoL, better quality of care with less aggressive end-of-life care, and decreased emotional distress for patients and their families. The value of palliative care services has been demonstrated through many randomized controlled trials that have shown that outcomes included improved QoL for patients and their caregivers, satisfaction with care received and end-of-life care planning and communication, and a reduction in unwanted treatments to prolong life (Shepperd et al., 2016).

The SARS-CoV-2 virus (COVID-19) pandemic served as a catalyst to shift service delivery models from hospital-centric service provision to care at home to reduce transmission of the virus. Although the links between rehabilitation professions and end-of-life care systems such as palliative care and hospice are often not clearly seen, it is important to focus on the elements that make up QoL and further examine the value that occupational therapy can bring to patients living with chronic illness and facing end-of-life.

Triple Aim

Donald Berwick, founder of the Institute for Health Care Improvement, launched the ***Triple Aim*** framework to promote better ways of providing health care while reducing growth in spending. Berwick et al. (2008) identified the Triple Aim goals as (1) improving the individual experience of care, (2) improving the health of populations, and (3) reducing the per capita costs of care for populations (p. 760). The Triple Aim served as a catalyst for health care reform during the Obama administration and has been a bridge for health care systems to shift to thinking about population health and pay closer attention to parts of the system where costs do not align with outcomes and patient satisfaction.

Palliative care programs, whether hospital or community based, are specifically designed to help patients cope more effectively with serious conditions while prioritizing QoL. Palliative care teams design and implement interventions that are targeted at helping patients and their families deal with the physical, emotional, and psychological issues related to their condition.

How Palliative Care Contributes to the Triple Aim

Palliative care originated in the United Kingdom, and in the early 1990s the modern U.S. palliative care model was born in academic medical centers that recognized that the core principles of hospice care should be applied to all patients with serious illness irrespective of their prognosis in an effort to improve their QoL (Morrison, 2013).

Palliative care programs are designed to help patients cope more effectively with serious and chronic conditions. Whether palliative care teams are hospital or community based, their approaches are similar. ***Palliative care teams*** often consist of physicians, nurses, social workers, chaplains, nutrition professionals, and more. The palliative care team initiates interventions designed to help patients deal with emotional and psychological issues related to their condition and provide medication to alleviate debilitating symptoms.

ENHANCING QUALITY OF LIFE

Research has shown that among patients using palliative care teams and supports, QoL was enhanced, symptom management improved, and patient satisfaction was greater. Caregivers' QoL also improved, and the burden of care lessened (Kavalieratos et al., 2016). Occupational therapy practitioners can show their distinct value by working with the patient to identify key areas of importance for enhanced QoL and by working with caregivers to identify ways to support their loved ones in this area.

IMPROVING HEALTH OUTCOMES

Palliative care has historically been seen as synonymous with end-of-life care, but discussion of how to best use this highly integrated approach to care earlier in the progression of disease coincides with the primary aim of improving patient outcomes (Oliver, 2018). Considering the links between the integration of care and improved patient outcomes, the WHO (2020) does not restrict palliative care to the end of life. Therefore, palliative care can be used earlier with patients as a means to enhance QoL and improve patient outcomes. Conversely, its definition of *palliative care* states that it is an approach that improves the QoL of patients and families facing the problems associated with a life-threatening illness through the prevention and relief of suffering and early identification and assessment and treatment of pain and other associated problems, including physical, psychosocial, and spiritual problems (WHO, 2020).

REDUCING COSTS

Palliative care has been found to be less costly relative to comparison groups (i.e., nonpalliative, traditional health care), and in most cases the difference in cost is statistically significant (Smith et al., 2014). However, it is important to note that models of palliative care and reimbursement vary widely across systems in the United States.

In addition, although it is an achievement that payers can now pay for palliative care, the modest reimbursement for a palliative care specialist evaluation and management and the inability to independently reimburse other palliative care team members skews the evidence for cost-effectiveness that is generated by an integrated interdisciplinary team working collaboratively to meet patients' needs. Therefore, to sustain the health care continuum, additional funding sources should be explored to ensure that the palliative care model can be maintained and patients can continue to receive highly integrated services that improve outcomes and satisfaction.

It is important to note that palliative care as outlined by the WHO (2020) includes a range of services delivered by an integrated network of professionals with equally important roles to play in support of the patient and their family: physicians, nurses, support professionals, paramedics, pharmacists, therapists, and volunteers.

How Hospice Contributes to the Triple Aim

In the 1950s a physician by the name of Dame Cicely Saunders recognized that specialized care for dying patients was necessary as Dr. Saunders and her team set out to link pain and symptom control to compassionate care. The concept moved its way across the pond in 1963 when Dr. Saunders was invited to speak on specialized care for the dying at Yale University. The path to where that care is today has been long, but in 1982, after numerous attempts, the hospice benefit was created within Medicare. Over the years, this service line has improved the end-of-life experience for both patients and their loved ones in countless ways. Today, although it is still underused, hospice is continuing to expand its integration into the U.S. health care system.

Hospice began as a demonstration program to study alternative health care delivery models, but it continues to be an exemplar of the kind of care people want their loved ones to receive at the end of life and want to receive themselves. Hospice is a value-based person-centered model of care that works to meet the needs of patients and their loved ones by addressing all aspects of a patient's well-being, including physical and emotional health, spiritual needs, family support, and comfort measures (Buck, 2011).

ENHANCING QUALITY OF LIFE

The foundation of hospice care is centered on the care, comfort, and QoL of a person with a terminal illness in their end-of-life transition. Therefore, the link between hospice care and enhanced QoL for a person at the end of life is easily identifiable in the literature. Although hospice care is known to be associated with improved symptom management and enhanced QoL, timely referrals are a common barrier to patients entering hospice care. Longer hospice utilization is directly correlated with increased quality of care, better pain and breathing management, and carrying out the patient's end-of-life wishes (Kumar et al., 2017).

IMPROVING HEALTH OUTCOMES

In thinking about the health care system's efficiency, it is important to remember family members' role in supporting their loved ones in hospice. Proper education of family members on how to contact the hospice nurse if a loved one begins to struggle is critical to avoid unnecessary and unwanted trips to the emergency department, and it is a precursor to enhancing QoL for the patient and also reducing health care costs. The ***Mobile Integrated Healthcare Community Paramedicine program*** is a health care delivery model innovation that leverages health care practitioners to provide high-quality patient-centered care to patients in their homes while reducing costs to the system overall (Xie et al., 2021). These programs have demonstrated improved health outcomes for hospice patients at home, allowing a decrease in paramedic transportation of hospice patients to the emergency department and providing continued support for family members (Breyre et al., 2022).

REDUCING COSTS

Approximately 25% of health care dollars are reported as wasteful spending (Shrank et al., 2019). IOM identifies six areas of wasteful spending, including (1) overtreatment, (2) failures of care coordination, (3) failures in the execution of care processes, (4) administrative complexity, (5) pricing failures, and (6) fraud and abuse (Berwick & Hackbarth, 2012). The extent to which hospice can reduce this spending is still under review. However, Aldridge et al.'s (2022) retrospective review demonstrated that enrollment in hospice among community-dwelling Medicare beneficiaries was associated with significantly lower costs in the last 3 days to 3 months of life, with no evidence that the cost was inadvertently shifted to families, who also reported significantly lower out-of-pocket costs in that same time period.

Quadruple Aim

The Triple Aim introduced by Donald Berwick and colleagues (2008) has rapidly spread as a means of optimizing the health care system to enhance QoL, improve health outcomes, and reduce overall costs. This concept has been embraced and utilized by many parts of the U.S. health care system. In their work with clinicians, Bodenheimer and Sinsky (2014) discovered that the stressful work life of health care professionals and staff affects their ability to achieve the Triple Aim. The addition of a fourth element—improving the work life of health care professionals and staff to improve population health overall—has often been referred to as the ***Quadruple Aim*** (Bodenheimer & Sinsky, 2014).

Concerns about health care staff burnout are well founded, according to a recent survey by Kirzinger et al. (2021), which found that 55% of frontline health care workers reported mental and physical exhaustion as a result of chronic workplace stress. This finding, along with other data, is alarming. The U.S. Department of Health and Human Services (2022) projects a shortage of more than 3 million essential health care professionals and 14,000 physicians by 2033.

Compassion fatigue is often common among health care professionals reporting high levels of stress. Sorenson et al. (2016) used the term ***compassion fatigue*** to describe the exhaustion that results from prolonged exposure to compassion stress among those who work in a caring profession, such as health professionals. Health care professionals often experience compassion fatigue and burnout when they know clinically what is in their patients' best interests, but barriers exist to providing high-quality care, whether as a result of others' lack of awareness and knowledge, systematic issues, or other contradictory factors. Here, advanced care planning can be an avenue not only to improving the quality of care but also to reducing health care costs, improving the health of populations, and reducing stress for the health care professional workforce.

Role of Advanced Care Planning

The National Academy of Medicine (2015) referred to ***advanced care planning*** as the whole process of discussion of the end of life, clarification of related values and goals, and embodiment of preferences through written documents and medical orders. The process can start at any time, should be revisited at regular intervals, and becomes more focused when a patient is having a health status change. Advanced care planning helps patients align the care they receive with their personal goals and values, therefore significantly improving their experience with the health care system (Bischoff et al., 2018).

Evidence also supports that advanced care planning improves the health of populations by increasing both quality and length of life. One example is a study by Neergaard et al. (2020) that concluded that, among seriously ill patients, those who had participated in advanced care planning had a 16% higher 1-year survival rate than those without advanced care plans. Advanced care planning has also been proven to reduce health care utilization, according to Klingler et al. (2016), and therefore to significantly decrease costs by helping patients and their family members avoid unnecessary, unwanted care, specifically when they do not opt for life-sustaining treatments.

Advanced care planning also has benefits for health care professionals because of its potential to increase health professional satisfaction and employee well-being and support a workforce that feels a lack of empowerment to improve their patients' QoL. For example, offering health plans that reward people for healthy behaviors, including an advanced care plan, is an effective way of aligning health care provider culture with the behaviors the organization seeks to foster in the patient population (Sikka et al., 2015). This also provides an opportunity for workforce education on advanced care planning and for the lived experience of being able to drive the plan in collaboration with the primary care team and families, and it facilitates an enhanced understanding of and comfort with having similar conversations with patients and their families.

Palliative Care and Hospice Education and Training Act: Including Occupational Therapy

The 2019–2020 ***Palliative Care and Hospice Education and Training Act*** (PCHETA; H.R. 647) is legislation to amend the Public Health Service Act (1944) to increase the number of permanent faculty in palliative care at accredited allopathic and osteopathic medical schools, nursing schools, social work programs, and other programs, including physician assistant programs, to promote education and research in palliative care and hospice.

At the time of publication, this legislation is awaiting reintroduction in the 118th Congress. It outlines that the U.S. Department of Health and Human Services should (1) provide palliative medicine and hospice academic career awards to people to promote their career development, (2) support entities that operate a palliative care and hospice education center, (3) support people in specified fields who are pursuing an advanced degree in palliative care or related fields, and (4) award grants to nursing programs to train people to provide palliative care.

PCHETA focuses on the education and training of physicians, nurses, social workers, and physician assistants in their efforts to increase awareness of the role of palliative and hospice care as well as advanced planning. This provides an opportunity for the occupational therapy profession to advocate for inclusion as part of PCHETA and to use its holistic lens as a part of the integrated care team and network to support advanced care planning with patients and their families.

Occupational Therapy Professionals as Advocates

Although occupational therapy may not be the first profession that comes to mind when thinking about palliative care, hospice care, or advanced care planning, it is important to examine the ways in which the lens through which practitioners see the patient and their environment is a valuable part of the conversation. Advocacy entails persuading people who matter to care about your issue (Daly, 2012).

KNOW YOUR VALUE

Occupational therapy professionals in palliative care and hospice address patients' physical and psychosocial needs, identifying their valued occupations and the barriers that limit participation (American Occupational Therapy Association, 2016). The occupational therapy lens is helpful in facilitating novel ways of thinking and doing for patients and their support system, despite the ongoing challenges and changes related to the disease process. These are fundamental positions practitioners can hold as they advocate for the inclusion of occupational therapy in palliative care and hospice education centers.

FORM ALLIANCES

With all advocacy comes the need for alliances. Occupational therapy practitioners can search out the gatekeepers who control access to the population, its decision makers, or both (Daly, 2012). In thinking about who can support occupational therapy in moving forward in the areas of palliative care and hospice, practitioners should intentionally reach out and develop networks with organizations such as the ***Center to Advance Palliative Care,*** a national organization dedicated to increasing the availability of quality, equitable health care for people with serious illnesses. It provides health professionals, such as occupational therapy practitioners, with training, tools, and assistance to meet their patients' needs. The American Academy of Hospice and Palliative Medicine (AAHPM; n.d.) is a professional organization for physicians, nurses, and health professionals seeking to advance awareness and integration of hospice and palliative care. A key part of the AAHPM strategic platform is to develop a diverse workforce that includes clinicians, educators, researchers, and innovators to extend the reach of and improve access to high-quality palliative and hospice care.

CREATE PERSUASIVE MESSAGES

It is essential that, as advocates for palliative and hospice care, occupational therapy practitioners understand how decisions are made. It is critical to know who the decision makers are and build a network of allies who can support occupational therapy's inclusion at the table. For example, practitioners can meet with their federal elected officials to request support for the PCHETA legislation and request the inclusion of occupational therapy. Simultaneously, they can meet with association leaders of those currently recognized in PCHETA to discuss the value that occupational therapy can bring to the team and the clients they serve to garner support for including occupational therapy in the act. Practitioners can share the stories of patients who have been helped by occupational therapy in palliative care and hospice to shine a light on the value the profession's contributions make in this part of the health care continuum.

As practitioners begin to explore the landscape that surrounds palliative care and hospice, it is important to identify who is likely to support its inclusion:

- Who might probable opponents be?
- What, if any, do these people have in terms of preconceptions about the message?
- Who will be affected by occupational therapy's inclusion?
- What needs do health professionals in the palliative care and hospice workforce have and how might occupational therapy fill the gap?

Once the decision makers and their perceptions are understood, occupational therapy practitioners can better show how the inclusion of occupational therapy in palliative care and hospice teams can be an asset to patients, their families, other health professionals, and organizations. In addition, the field can lift the voices of those who are not at the table. Evidence is an important and vital part of the advocacy effort. Of equal importance is bringing forward the stories of patients whose QoL was enhanced because occupational therapy was part of the palliative care or hospice team. Evidence pulls decision makers in to hear more, but the story and lived experiences of others will most often inspire them to take action. Prove occupational therapy's value by using good evidence, including the meaningful stories of those in the field and those on the receiving end of rehabilitation in palliative and hospice care (Daly, 2012).

Summary

For occupational therapy practitioners seeking to make a difference in the QoL of patients and their families, palliative care and hospice hold opportunities to support meaningful engagement in occupations. As practitioners continue to explore the distinct value occupational therapy can contribute to patients and their families in palliative care and hospice, they can also consider ways to advocate for what occupational therapy can contribute to improve the patient experience, improve outcomes, and reduce costs to the health care system.

Amy J. Lamb, OTD, OTR/L, FAOTA, is the CLO/founder of Meraki & Me, where she provides executive leadership development coaching services. She is the past-president of the American Occupational Therapy Association (2016–1019) and Chair of AOTPAC (2006–2012). She is a teaching professional in Boston University's postprofessional OTD program, where she brings with her the valuable combination of clinical practice as a licensed occupational therapist and health care policy experience at the state and federal levels.

REFERENCES

Aldridge, M. D., Moreno, J., McKendrick, K., Li, L., Brody, A., & May, P. (2022). Association between hospice enrollment and total health care costs for insurers and families, 2002–2018. *JAMA Health Forum, 3*(2), e215104. https://doi.org/10.1001/jamahealthforum.2021.5104

American Academy of Hospice and Palliative Medicine. (n.d.). *AAHPM and the specialty of hospice and palliative medicine.* https://aahpm.org/about/about

American Occupational Therapy Association. (2016). Role of occupational therapy in end-of-life care. *American Journal of Occupational Therapy, 70*(Suppl. 2), 7012410075. https://doi.org/10.5014/ajot.2016.706S17

Berwick, D. M., & Hackbarth, A. D. (2012). Eliminating waste in US health care. *JAMA, 307*(14), 1513–1516. https://doi.org/10.1001/jama.2012.362

Berwick, D. M., Nolan, T. W., & Whittington, J. (2008). The Triple Aim: Care, health, and cost. *Health Affairs, 27,* 759–769. https://doi.org/10.1377/hlthaff.27.3.759

Bischoff, K., O'Riordan, D., Marks, A., Sudore, R., & Pantilat, S. Z. (2018). Care planning for inpatients referred for palliative care consultation. *JAMA Internal Medicine, 178*(1), 48–54. https://doi.org/10.1001/jamainternmed.2017.6313

Bodenheimer, T., & Sinsky, C. (2014). From Triple to Quadruple Aim: Care of the patient requires care of the provider. *Annals of Family Medicine, 12,* 573–576. https://doi.org/10.1370/afm.1713

Breyre, A., Taigman, M., Salvucci, A., & Sporer, K. (2022). Effect of a mobile integrated hospice healthcare program on emergency medical services transport to the emergency department. *Prehospital Emergency Care, 26,* 364–369. https://doi.org/10.1080/10903127.2021.1900474

Buck, J. (2011). Policy and the reformation of hospice: Lessons from the past for the future of palliative care. *Journal of Hospice and Palliative Nursing, 13*(6), S35–S43. https://doi.org/10.1097/NJH.0b013e3182331160

Center for Improving Value in Health Care. (2012). *Palliative care best practices: A guide for long-term care and hospice.* https://www.capc.org/documents/download/947/

Center to Advance Palliative Care. (2023). *Welcome to the Center to Advance Palliative Care.* https://www.capc.org/

Cohn, J., Corrigan, J., Lynn, J., Meier, D., Miller, J., Shega, J., & Wang, S. (2017). Community-based models of care delivery for people with serious illness [discussion paper]. *NAM Perspectives.* https://doi.org/10.31478/201704b

Daly, J. (2012). *Advocacy: Championing ideas and influencing others.* Yale University Press.

Heo, D. S., Yoo, S. H., Keam, B., Yoo, K., Choi, I., & Kim, M. J. (2022). Hospice-palliative medicine as a model of value-based healthcare. *Journal of Korean Medical Science, 37,* e111. https://doi.org/10.3346/jkms.2022.37.e111

Hughes, M. T., & Smith, T. J. (2014). The growth of palliative care in the United States. *Annual Review of Public Health, 35,* 459–475. https://doi.org/10.1146/annurev-publhealth-032013-182406

Institute of Medicine. (2015). *Dying in America: Improving quality and honoring individual preferences near the end of life.* The National Academies Press. https://doi.org/10.17226/18748

Joynt, K. E., Figueroa, J. F., Beaulieu, N., Wild, R. C., Orav, E. J., & Jha, A. K. (2017). Segmenting high-cost Medicare patients into potentially actionable cohorts. *Healthcare, 5,* 62–67. https://doi.org/10.1016/j.hjdsi.2016.11.002.

Kavalieratos, D., Corbelli, J., Zhang, D., Dionne-Odom, N., Ernecoff, N. C., Hanmer, J., . . . Schenker, Y. (2016). Association between palliative care and patient and caregiver outcomes: A systematic review and meta-analysis. *JAMA, 316,* 2104–2114. https://doi.org/10.1001/jama.2016.16840

Kirzinger, A., Kearney, A., Hamel, L., & Brodie, M. (2021, April 6). *KFF/The Washington Post Frontline Health Care Workers Survey.* Kaiser Family Foundation.

https://www.kff.org/report-section/kff-the-washington-post-frontline-health-care-workers-survey-toll-of-the-pandemic/

Klingler, C., in der Schmitten, J., & Marckmann, G. (2016). Does facilitated advance care planning reduce the costs of care near the end of life? Systematic review and ethical considerations. *Palliative Medicine, 30,* 423–433. https://doi.org/10.1177/0269216315601346

Kumar, P., Wright, A. A., Hatfield, L. A., Temel, J. S., & Keating, N. L. (2017). Family perspectives on hospice care experiences of patients with cancer. *Journal of Clinical Oncology, 35,* 432–439. https://doi.org/10.1200/JCO.2016.68.9257

Morrison, R. S. (2013). Models of palliative care delivery in the United States. *Current Opinion in Supportive and Palliative Care, 7,* 201–206. https://doi.org/10.1097/SPC.0b013e32836103e5

National Academies of Sciences, Engineering, and Medicine. (2016). *Families caring for an aging America.* The National Academies Press. https://doi.org/10.17226/23606

National Academy of Medicine. (2015). *Dying in America: Improving quality and honoring individual preferences near the end of life.* National Academies Press.

Neergaard, M. A., Skorstengaard, M. H., Brogaard, T., Bendstrup, E., Løkke, A., Aagaard, S., . . . Jensen, A. B. (2020). Advance care planning and longer survival in the terminally ill: A randomised controlled trial unexpected finding. *BMJ Supportive and Palliative Care, 10,* 221–222. https://doi.org/10.1136/bmjspcare-2019-001906

Oliver, D. (2018). Improving patient outcomes through palliative care integration in other specialised health services: What we have learned so far and how can we improve? *Annals of Palliative Medicine, 7*(Suppl. 3), S219–S230. https://doi.org/10.21037/apm.2018.05.05

Palliative Care and Hospice Education and Training Act, H.R. 647, 116th Congress (2019–2020). https://www.congress.gov/bill/116th-congress/house-bill/647

Patient Protection and Affordable Care Act, Pub. L. 111-148, 42 U.S.C. §§ 18001–18121 (2010).

Public Health Service Act, 42 U.S.C. 201 *et seq.* (1944).

Shepperd, S., Goncalves-Bradley, D. C., Straus, S. E., & Wee, B. (2016). Hospital at home: Home-based end-of-life care. *Cochrane Database of Systematic Reviews.* https://doi.org/10.1002/14651858.CD009231.pub2

Shrank, W. H., Rogstad, T. L., & Parekh, N. (2019). Waste in the US health care system: Estimated costs and potential for savings. *JAMA, 322,* 1501–1509. https://doi.org/10.1001/jama.2019.13978

Sikka, R., Morath, J. M., & Leape, L. (2015). The Quadruple Aim: Care, health, cost and meaning in work. *BMJ Quality and Safety, 24,* 608–610. https://doi.org/10.1136/bmjqs-2015-004160

Smith, S., Brick, A., O'Hara, S., & Normand C. (2014). Evidence on the cost and cost-effectiveness of palliative care: A literature review. *Palliative Medicine, 28,* 130–150. https://doi.org/10.1177/0269216313493466

Sorenson, C., Bolick, B., Wright, K., & Hamilton, R. (2016). Understanding compassion fatigue in healthcare providers: A review of current literature. *Journal of Nursing Scholarship, 48,* 456–465. https://doi.org/10.1111/jnu.12229

U.S. Department of Health and Human Services. (2022, May 23). *New Surgeon General advisory sounds alarm on health worker burnout and resignation* [Press release]. https://www.hhs.gov/about/news/2022/05/23/new-surgeon-general-advisory-sounds-alarm-on-health-worker-burnout-and-resignation.html

Warraich, H. J., Hernandez, A. F., & Allen, L. A. (2017). How medicine has changed the end of life for patients with cardiovascular disease. *Journal of the American College of Cardiology, 70,* 1276–1289. https://doi.org/10.1016/j.jacc.2017.07.735

World Health Organization. (2020). *Palliative care.* https://www.who.int/news-room/fact-sheets/detail/palliative-care.

World Health Organization. (2023). *WHOQOL: Measuring quality of life.* https://www.who.int/tools/whoqol

Xie, F., Yan, J., Agarwal, G., & Ferron, R. (2021). Economic analysis of mobile integrated health care delivered by emergency medical services paramedic teams. *JAMA Network Open, 4*(2), e210055. https://doi.org/10.1001/jamanetworkopen.2021.0055

2

Demonstrating Occupational Therapy's Distinct Value: Chronic Conditions and Terminal Illness

ANN B. BEST, MHS, OTR/L

Learning Objectives

After completing this chapter, readers will be able to

- explain how occupational therapy practitioners serve many patients with chronic conditions or terminal illness in settings in which they are already practicing,
- identify opportunities and strategies to improve quality of life (QoL) by addressing the often unmet needs of this population and their caregivers, and
- use a road map for QoL and habilitative work that leads to palliative or hospice care.

Key Terms and Concepts

caregiver burden
chronic illness
chronic pain management
Clinical Assessment of Modes
decision-making algorithms
diversity, equity, and inclusion
empathy
fatigue management
functional maintenance programs
habilitation

health equity
Intentional Relationship Model
management of disease-specific symptoms
mind–body self-care
occupational therapy road map
Patient Protection and Affordable Care Act
Quadruple Aim
quality of life
Quintuple Aim
rabbit effect
sleep hygiene
Spoon Theory
therapeutic use of self
transgenerational trauma
trauma processing
trauma-informed care
Triple Aim
Zen of therapy

Every day, occupational therapy practitioners are working as rehabilitative specialists with clients who have ***chronic illness,*** which includes "conditions that last 1 year or more and require ongoing medical attention or limit activities of daily living or both" (Centers for Disease Control and Prevention [CDC], 2022a). The number of people with chronic conditions is growing; it represents 60% of adults in the United States (CDC, 2021b, 2022a). According to the CDC (2021b), seven of these chronic diseases represent the leading causes of death and are a driver of the nation's health care costs: heart disease, cancer, chronic lung disease, stroke, Alzheimer's disease, diabetes, and chronic kidney disease.

Several factors have contributed to the increased prevalence and cost of chronic disease, including the "rising age of the population and disease-specific risk factors such as poor nutrition and sleep, tobacco use, lack of physical activity, and failure to attend annual health care visits. In effect, many adults with chronic disease experience disability" (Fields & Smallfield, 2022, p. 1).

Researchers are also finding that the caregivers of those with chronic conditions are at greater risk for lower quality of life (QoL) and greater physical and mental distress than their counterparts (Fields & Smallfield, 2022).

Although occupational therapy practitioners have the opportunity to treat people with chronic disease and their caregivers in any setting, a majority of practitioners work in settings that treat these people for the debility they experience because of the disease or the factors that led to the disease. Well over half of all practitioners surveyed recently work in hospitals, home health, and skilled nursing facilities (American Occupational Therapy Association [AOTA], 2019). These settings offer the health care and services that are necessary and ongoing for those with chronic conditions, as well as their caregivers, who may be experiencing conditions secondary to this role.

This chapter describes opportunities for occupational therapy practitioners to address unmet needs for those with chronic illness and their caregivers. Included is the rationale and supporting evidence of key strategies for work with clients, their caregivers, and the interprofessional team. Areas of focus include therapeutic use of self to improve ***QoL,*** which is a person's perception of well-being in all aspects of their life. The chapter also discusses environmental enhancements to establish social connections and community and habilitation to improve engagement in occupation.

Occupational Therapy Treatment of Chronic Illness: Current Focus

Health care priorities for the United States were visualized in the ***Triple Aim*** framework. In 2006, researchers at the Institute for Healthcare Improvement (IHI; 2022) designed this framework with the core intentions of (1) improving patient experience, (2) improving population health, and (3) reducing costs. It coincides with AOTA's (2017) *Vision 2025* that "occupational therapy maximizes health, well-being, and quality of life for all people, populations, and communities through effective solutions that facilitate participation in everyday living" (p. 1). Ongoing shifts in health care policy related to reimbursement, referral procedures in treatment settings, and limited time for advocacy by occupational therapy practitioners have resulted in unmet needs for those with chronic disease (Baxter et al., 2017; Fields & Smallfield, 2022; Rafeedie et al., 2018). Theories and frames of reference that support maintaining engagement in occupation when chronic conditions and disease processes are causing a steady decline in client factors and performance skills are well rooted in occupational therapy education. However, in reality, practitioners have not always been adequately equipped to use this approach despite policy and support by AOTA. For rehabilitation specialists, a large majority of occupational therapy treatment is focused on outcomes of improvement in client factors and performance skills related to occupational performance versus maintaining participation in occupation (Rafeedie et al., 2018). It seems the hands of the profession have encountered barriers to what its heart and mind prescribe for this population.

Opportunities To Address Needs

FUNCTIONAL MAINTENANCE PROGRAMS

Most chronic diseases cause either a gradual decline in function or involve episodes of exacerbation and remission with episodic decline in function; people with either would benefit from skilled therapy to establish and use ***functional maintenance programs*** (FMPs), which are designed to maintain current functional levels while preventing further loss of function with focus on outcomes of QoL, participation, and wellness. Maintenance programs have been available through Medicare but are not widely used (Rafeedie et al., 2018). In 2013, the Jimmo et al. versus Sebelius settlement resulted in the clarification that therapy services should indeed be considered skilled in instances when prevention of decline, not progress, is the goal (Centers for Medicare & Medicaid Services [CMS], 2021a, 2021b). Limited knowledge and support of these services and certain restrictions, such as that the services had to be provided by a therapist rather than an assistant, prevented widespread use of FMPs. Because of the work of therapy advocacy groups, CMS changed its policy to allow therapists to delegate this necessary service to an assistant (CMS, 2022). This is significant for clients who are dealing with chronic conditions because they will have greater access to skilled therapy services in skilled nursing facilities and home health and outpatient care. Skilled services were previously believed to be covered only if the benefactor showed improvement; now services that are necessary to prevent or slow further deterioration because of a chronic condition will be considered skilled.

For people with chronic illness, habilitative services become significant in teaching them new ways to connect socially and with the community and to participate in meaningful daily living skills in a new and different manner. "Habilitative services and devices help a person keep, learn, or improve skills or functioning for daily living" (AOTA et al., 2021, p. 1). Baxter et al. (2017) described a lack of survivorship care for cancer survivors that can also be true for survivors of chronic conditions. Evidence has shown that these survivors experience a loss of self-efficacy, independence, activity, and participation that ultimately affects their ability to participate in employment, education, and social connections (Baxter et al., 2017). These limitations can be addressed by occupational therapy practitioners with habilitation of new skills to deal with symptoms of pain, fatigue, and weakness and adaptations to enable participation in daily living and social pursuits. Fields and Smallfield's (2022) *Occupational Therapy Practice Guidelines for Adults With Chronic Conditions* provide strategies to address QoL and participation issues for this population. Habilitation of self-management skills through education, goal setting, and problem solving over an extended time with follow-up to establish habits and routines is recommended.

CARE FOR THE CAREGIVER

One of the core factors of success with maintenance programs is caregiver education and follow-through. However, as noted by Novak and Jewell (2020), inadequate follow-through is frequent. Health care providers are experiencing burnout, and caregivers of those with chronic disease have lower life satisfaction and decreased health. The IHI thus added a new dimension—workforce well-being and safety—to the Triple Aim to address the high level of burnout, fatigue, and stress of health care providers, naming it the ***Quadruple Aim*** (Bodenheimer & Sinsky, 2014; Nundy et al., 2022; Rafeedie et al., 2018). Occupational therapy can provide resources for health care providers by expanding services to address relationship building, physical care, and emotional support of caregivers.

EQUITABLE ACCESS THROUGH PRIMARY CARE

Health equity is "the state in which everyone has a fair and just opportunity to attain their highest level of health" (CDC, 2022b). It is part of what is being called the ***Quintuple Aim*** (Nundy et al., 2022) and is based on the need for improved access to health care for all. The World Health Organization (WHO) recognized the need to prioritize universal access to rehabilitation because of the presence of comorbid chronic conditions in the world's aging population; it declared that function should be the third health indicator, along with mortality and morbidity (Heinemann et al., 2020). The 2010 ***Patient Protection and Affordable Care Act*** (ACA; P. L. 111-148) "mandates marketplace health plans to cover essential health benefits, including habilitation and rehabilitation services. However, services vary greatly as a result of variations in individual state and federal interpretations of the ACA" (Baxter et al., 2017, p. 4). Although services are recognized as significant, they are not being provided to meet the needs of chronically ill people in an equitable manner. Since passage of the ACA, the focus of primary and acute care has shifted to ongoing management of chronic conditions, and occupational therapy practitioners should be key team members in providing access to the habilitation services needed by people who are chronically ill (AOTA, 2020d; Leland et al., 2017; Murphy et al., 2017; Rouch et al., 2022; Stern, 2019). Rouch et al. (2022) showed that the contributions of therapists working in primary care to positive outcomes included "working with patients on self-management, functional problem solving and behavioral change" (p. 1) and that much of their work entailed managing chronic conditions.

Strategies To Improve Quality of Life

Occupational therapists can address needs and support clients and their caregivers to engage in meaningful occupations from birth to death. The profession's philosophy, theories, models, and frames of reference provide evidence-based practice guidelines to improve the QoL of those experiencing chronic illness and their caregivers, as well as the health care providers who serve them. Core strategies and techniques should be embedded throughout the occupational therapy process, particularly in therapeutic use of self, with an increased focus on care for the caregiver; environmental factors related to social connection; and implementation of habilitation for self-management.

THERAPEUTIC USE OF SELF

A cornerstone of all occupational therapy intervention is therapeutic use of self (AOTA, 2020b). It is considered a crucial element in influencing client outcomes (AOTA, 2020b; Seymour, 2012). AOTA (2020b) describes ***therapeutic use of self*** as the part of the occupational therapy process "in which occupational therapy practitioners develop and manage their therapeutic relationship with clients by using professional reasoning, empathy, and a client-centered, collaborative approach to service delivery" (p. 20).

Early (2017) described foundational qualities of therapeutic use of self as including empathy, sensitivity, respect, genuineness, warmth, humor, self-disclosure, specificity, immediacy, and collaboration. Early work by Weinstein (1998) explored therapeutic use of self and "elements of artful practice of therapists in mental health settings" and found three prevailing themes: "therapeutic work as a vehicle for healing, collaborative guidance, and the Zen of therapy" (p. 579). The ***Zen of therapy*** was termed by one study participant as a mystical connection between therapist and patient:

> The client is somehow touched by the therapist's authentic presence, even if the therapist has not intervened and no words or activity have been shared. There is a sense of spaciousness and accommodation. The situation can be quite ordinary yet engender a sense of mystery and magic. (Weinstein, 1998, p. 583)

The ***rabbit effect,*** a term coined by Harding (2019), came from an experiment with rabbits in 1978 showing the relationship between heart health and a high-fat diet. It found that the kindness provided by a lab assistant reversed much of the negative impact of the high-fat diet on her group of rabbits. "Take a rabbit with an unhealthy lifestyle. Talk to it. Hold it. Give it affection. And many adverse effects of diet disappear. The relationship made a difference" (Harding, 2019, p. i).

Taylor's (2008) work conceptualizes therapeutic use of self as an intentional relationship established during the therapeutic process. The ***Intentional Relationship Model*** was developed to provide a framework for this relationship; it describes six therapeutic communication "modes": (1) advocating, (2) collaborating, (3) empathizing, (4) encouraging, (5) instructing, and (6) problem solving (Taylor, 2008). Significant to therapeutic use of self is the ability to shift one's personality and communication style to fit the needs of a social demand by the client, caregiver, or interdisciplinary team member. "In the Empathizing mode, therapists strive to understand clients' thoughts and feelings by validating their emotions through nonjudgmental statements"; further research established that "this mode was highly correlated with clients' motivation toward occupation and overall participation in rehabilitation" (Fan & Taylor, 2018, p. 1). Brown (2013) quantified qualities of empathy in her work, describing ***empathy*** as feeling with someone that fuels connection. She described attributes of empathy as kindness, curiosity, connecting and listening, understanding the feeling, and allowing opportunities for second chances to get it right (O'Brien, 2019; Stuart, 2020).

When working with people with chronic illness, it is important that the same strategies of therapeutic use of self used with clients be applied to connections with caregivers and interdisciplinary team members. Occupational therapy's domain and process, practice guidelines, and literature support the impact of therapeutic use of self on client outcomes and addresses the need for caregiver and interdisciplinary work. Caregivers are the drivers of the success of maintenance programs (Novak & Jewell, 2020), so occupational therapy practitioners should work to establish and improve their connections with caregivers through these same strategies during frequent and ongoing meetings.

If there is a disconnect between the occupational therapy practitioner's and client's or caregiver's perception of a needed communication style or therapeutic use of self, then there is the potential for feelings of "disrespect and disempowerment in therapy" (Fan et al., 2022). Fan et al. (2022) demonstrated that such a disconnect indeed occurred at times when clients perceived that therapists were communicating by instructing and therapists perceived they were communicating by empathizing (Fan et al., 2022). It is as important to ensure that the therapist's and client's or caregiver's communication style match. Similar to Chapman's (2010) *The Five Love Languages,* a book and model that help partners improve relationships by understanding each other's ways of expressing and receiving love, therapists need to take time to really listen and observe the receiver's response. Assessment measures such as the ***Clinical Assessment of Modes*** can help to ensure a good fit, but most important is the "clinicians' development of a flexible therapeutic style, congruent with their personality and their clients' needs" and understanding of the client's or caregiver's past experiences and relevant impact (Fan et al., 2022, p. 5).

Past experiences of stress and trauma can affect therapeutic use of self and social connection. Literature shows that people who have experienced stressful or traumatic experiences are at greater risk for medical and mental health conditions. The landmark Adverse Childhood Experiences (ACEs) study (CDC, 2021a) and later research demonstrated the direct correlation between the number of ACEs and chronic health conditions, specifically heart disease, stroke, liver disease, lung cancer, chronic obstructive pulmonary disease, skeletal injuries, and autoimmune disorders (Fette et al., 2019; Grossman et al., 2021). Moreover, diagnosis and treatment of chronic health conditions have potential to retraumatize (Grossman et al., 2021). Finally, trauma can be transgenerational; even if trauma was not personally experienced, the experience of a parent or grandparent can have an impact (DeAngelis, 2019; Lehrner & Yehuda, 2018).

The use of ***trauma-informed care*** to establish a social connection and during therapeutic use of self is imperative and promoted by health providers, as well as state and federal policymakers. It begins with the expectation and use of trauma-informed principles in a universal precaution–type manner. These principles align directly with the other strategies of therapeutic use of self, with an additional emphasis on providing an environment that is perceived as safe, as well as recognizing and providing support for symptoms of trauma stress (CDC, 2021a; Fette et al., 2019; Grossman et al., 2021).

Caregivers often experience trauma as a result of their role with chronically ill, injured, or dying loved ones, which, evidence shows, in turn results in decreased mental and physical health. ***Caregiver burden*** is the "physical, psychological, social, or economic strain that caregivers may experience during the care of a loved one" (Carmassi et al., 2020, p. 1). It occurs because of new and often unfamiliar responsibilities, along with an overwhelming sense of concern. Evidence suggests this burden sometimes results in psychological trauma (Carmassi et al., 2020). Carmassi et al. (2020) identified factors that decreased this impact on health, which included work outside of the home, supportive family and relationship with the patient, use of mindfulness and adaptive coping strategies, and a sense of control gained through education and active involvement with health care providers.

> Clinicians could indeed provide prompt effective support to caregivers by recognizing the magnitude of their perceived stress and by developing novel and effective supportive strategies. Developing guidelines for family-centered care and support in wards treating severely ill patients could help nourishing psychological wellbeing of caregivers and, possibly, of patients. (Carmassi et al., 2020, p. 12; see Exhibit 2.1)

Health care providers are also at risk for trauma associated with care for people who are chronically or terminally ill. Evidence has suggested that self-care strategies that can be easily incorporated in the workplace and supportive supervision at work were effective in improving health care providers' resiliency. Specific strategies found to be beneficial included

EXHIBIT 2.1.

KEY STRATEGIES OF THERAPEUTIC USE OF SELF TO IMPROVE QoL FOR CLIENTS, CAREGIVERS, AND INTERPROFESSIONAL TEAM MEMBERS

<table>
<tr><th colspan="2">Specific techniques to maximize the effectiveness of therapeutic use of self for clients, caregivers, and interdisciplinary team members</th></tr>
<tr><td>Empathizing and encouraging IRM communication mode: builds relationship, connection, and trust</td><td>
• Use kindness and show genuine concern (Harding, 2019).
• Practice perspective taking:
  ○ Stay out of judgment, including judging another person's pain or discounting their experience; refrain from comments that invalidate someone's experience or make them feel wrong
  ○ Recognize emotion—connect with the other's emotion by remembering experiencing it yourself
  ○ Communication—validate the other's feeling and experience with care and concern (Brown, 2013; O'Brien, 2019)
• Use primary and advanced accurate empathy techniques to better understand the client (Cole, 2018).
• Match another's personality tone and rhythm by connecting with those aspects of your own personality (Taylor, 2008).
• Assess perceptions of communication mode by using a tool such as the CAM to ensure satisfactory connection (Fan et al., 2022)
• Apply trauma-informed principles:
  ○ Provide physical and emotional safety through confidentiality and environmental supports.
  ○ Be trustworthy and transparent.
  ○ Be aware of and listen for cultural, historical, and gender issues.
</td></tr>
</table>

(Continued)

EXHIBIT 2.1.

KEY STRATEGIES OF THERAPEUTIC USE OF SELF TO IMPROVE QoL FOR CLIENTS, CAREGIVERS, AND INTERPROFESSIONAL TEAM MEMBERS *(Cont.)*

Instructing in and collaborating on IRM communication mode: increases success of habilitation or rehabilitation training	• Prioritize connection with caregivers and other health professionals to establish functional maintenance programming. • Apply trauma-informed principles: ○ Establish opportunities for peer support and mutual self-help with collaboration and mutuality.

Advocating IRM communication mode: improves support for and reimbursement of services	• Truly connect with interdisciplinary team members by supporting and encouraging their part of the care plan and using DEI strategies.
	• Provide documentation to payer sources to support maintenance and nontraditional rehabilitative services.
	• Apply trauma-informed principles:
	  ○ Provide opportunities for empowerment, voice, and choice.
	  ○ Provide support for cultural, historical, and gender issues.

Note. CAM = Clinical Assessment of Modes; DEI = diversity, equity, and inclusion; IRM = Intentional Relationship Model; QoL = quality of life.

self-management of mind–body skills (e.g., breathing, yoga, meditation), cognitive stress management strategies, and targeted professional development (Apostol et al., 2021; Perez et al., 2015; Soper, 2022). These are similar to the habilitation strategies that have been effective for self-management of clients with chronic illness and their caregivers.

ENVIRONMENTAL FACTORS: SUPPORT SOCIAL CONNECTION

Social connections are significant factors in health and QoL. Harding's (2019) rabbit effect entails hidden factors that bring about health: "factors like love, friendship, and dignity, [and] the designs of our neighborhoods, schools, and workplaces" (p. i; see Figure 2.1). Harding's abundance of evidence to support these hidden factors directly corresponds with occupational therapy philosophy. Included in Yerxa's (1992) description of the relevant health care history that brought about an increased awareness of these hidden factors is, interestingly, Dr. Adolph Meyer, who is considered "one of the first philosophers of occupational therapy" (p. 79). The significant evidence for the impact of social and environmental factors on QoL supports the incorporation of these strategies into work with chronically ill people and those who provide care to them (Rafeedie et al., 2018). As Martino et al. (2015) point out,

> From psychological theories to recent research, there is significant evidence that social support and feeling connected can help people maintain a healthy body mass index, control blood sugars, improve cancer survival, decrease cardiovascular mortality, decrease depressive symptoms, mitigate posttraumatic stress disorder symptoms, and improve overall mental health. The opposite of connection, social isolation, has a negative effect on health and can increase depressive symptoms as well as mortality. (p. 466)

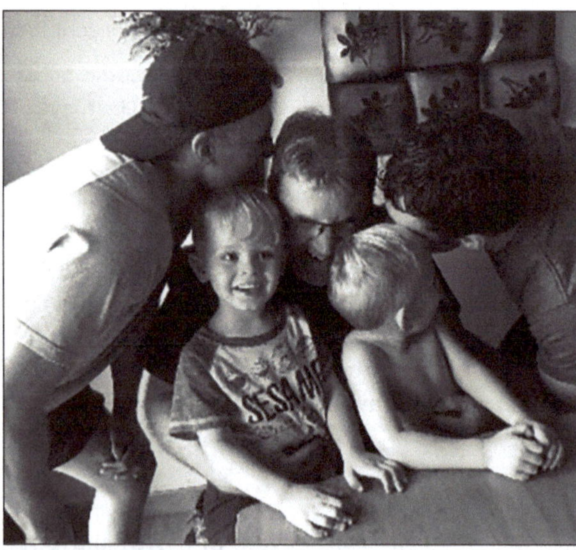

Figure 2.1 Social connection is significant in health and QoL.

Source. A. Best. Used with permission.

Occupational therapy practitioners can contribute to fueling social connection by analyzing environments, providing supports, and building social performance skills.

Diversity, equity, and inclusion (DEI) affect social connection. AOTA (2020c) provided a description of these concepts with their statement affirming "the inalienable right of every individual to feel welcomed, valued, a sense of belonging, and respected while accessing and participating in society, regardless of the internal or external factors that make every individual unique" (p. 1). Each person is *diverse* with "unique attributes, values, and beliefs" (AOTA, 2020c, p. 1), and individuals deserve *equity,* which is "access to the same opportunities, taking into consideration the advantages and disadvantages" one faces (AOTA, 2020c, p. 1), and *inclusion,* which is "acceptance and support of diversity wherein the uniqueness of beliefs, values, and attributes is welcomed, valued, and leveraged for maximum engagement" (AOTA, 2020c, p. 1). Client-centered care concepts, inherent in therapeutic use of self, would appear to allow full appreciation of the uniqueness of each person's cultural differences; however, barriers exist that range from apparent to invisible. Analysis and elimination of barriers can be difficult because of unconscious and implicit biases, perceptions, and misunderstandings.

In addition, ***transgenerational trauma*** may be present. Trauma can be transmitted to later generations and be experienced as discrimination stress, which has been shown to be associated with numerous physical and mental health problems (Kulig et al., 2013; Thoits, 2010). Improving awareness and DEI skill building will assist in achieving equity and eliminating barriers to inclusion for clients, support systems, and interprofessional team members (AOTA, 2020a). Because occupational therapy's domain allows a focus on relationship building through therapeutic use of self, practitioners are well poised to be the glue (Kelly, 2022) that facilitates the inclusion of everyone with whom they work (Exhibit 2.2).

Other barriers need to be overcome for caregivers of and health care providers working with chronically ill people. Social support has been identified as an important resiliency and coping factor for these groups; however, it is often missing (Apostol et al., 2021; Perez et al., 2015; Schoultz, 2021; Soper, 2022). A concentrated effort by occupational therapy to include caregivers in their work in providing supports for clients for social connectedness could meet this need (Exhibit 2.2).

EXHIBIT 2.2.
KEY STRATEGIES FOR PROVIDING ENVIRONMENTAL ENHANCEMENTS TO ESTABLISH SOCIAL CONNECTION AND COMMUNITY

Analyzing context and providing supports to clients and caregivers	• Analyze environment and context for client participation in social events or situations, and identify barriers and provide adaptive equipment or compensatory strategies to allow participation. • Provide adequate supports or eliminate barriers related to equity and inclusion.
Addressing social performance skills	• Offer scaffolding to build skills. • Analyze the need for and provide adaptive equipment and techniques.
Connecting with and valuing others	• Provide caregivers with opportunities to connect with other caregivers or support groups; assist in providing respite care. • Increase knowledge of and skills for understanding and handling implicit or unconscious bias, microaggressions, and difficult conversations.
Advocating for equity	• Connect with clients' primary care physicians. o Establish an ongoing relationship to provide prevention and self-management before decline occurs.

HABILITATION THROUGH MAINTENANCE PROGRAMS

Self-management

Occupational therapy intervention approaches can be ideal for the necessary habilitation of self-maintenance skills to affect QoL of people with chronic illness and their caregivers (Figure 2.2). Unique to occupational therapy are interventions for teaching and doing, which allows for cognitive appreciation and kinesthetic learning of techniques. The profession also has within its domain work with performance patterns that allows for the establishment of habits and routines and

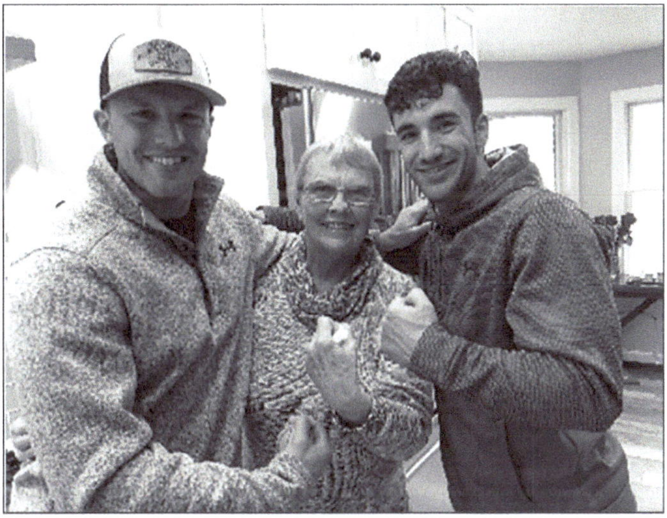

Figure 2.2 Successful use of self-management strategies results in a perception of strength, which enables increased participation in meaningful activities.

Source. A. Best. Used with permission.

ensures follow-through (Fields & Smallfield, 2022; Stern 2019). The literature provides ample evidence of the effectiveness of self-management strategies used by the profession with clients with chronic illness (see Table 2.1).

Themes that emerge on the basis of the evidence for self-management of chronic disease relate to mind–body self-care, management of disease-specific symptoms, chronic pain management, fatigue management, sleep hygiene, and trauma processing and resiliency training with sensory modulation. ***Mind–body self-care*** is a holistic approach to managing the physical, psychological, and social impacts of disease (Fields & Smallfield, 2022). ***Management of disease-specific symptoms*** is targeted to specific diagnoses and the related symptoms that occur, and it includes techniques such as foot care and dietary changes, with blood sugar monitoring for those with diabetes, fatigue management for those with heart disease and chronic obstructive pulmonary disease, and activity and trigger management for those with asthma and kidney disease (Fields & Smallfield, 2022; Smallfield et al., 2021).

TABLE 2.1. Key Habilitative Services to Improve QoL and Engagement in Occupation

Theme	Examples
	Self-management
Mind–body self-care	• Sleep hygiene, nutrition, physical activity, and relaxation techniques • Group supports (Fields & Smallfield, 2022)
Management of disease-specific symptoms	• "Foot care self-management education (e.g., foot self-care, risk factors, hygiene, footwear, prevention, goal setting, problem solving), in addition to usual care, for adults with diabetes" (Fields & Smallfield, 2022, p. 4) • Fatigue management for people with COPD and heart disease • Dietary changes and self-monitoring—individual and group sessions and follow-up for people with diabetes, decreased cholesterol levels and BMI for people with hypertension • Diagnosis education and self-treatment and trigger management for people with asthma or chronic kidney disease • Physical activity for people with heart disease and COPD—aerobic exercise and resistance training to improve ADL performance (Fields & Smallfield, 2022)
Chronic pain management	• Mindfulness, relaxation, and breathing techniques • Biofeedback • Chronic pain education • Neutral spine education for ADLs, IADLs, and sleep and rest; functional transfer training • Supports for comfort positioning • Therapeutic touch and massage • Self-myofascial release techniques, the Melt Method (Hitzman, 2016) • Fall prevention training • Ergonomics, body mechanics, and joint protection

(Continued)

TABLE 2.1. Key Habilitative Services to Improve QoL and Engagement in Occupation *(Cont.)*

Theme	Examples
	• Adaptive equipment and compensatory strategies for ADLs and IADLs • Self-expressive activities • Self-efficacy and advocacy • Medication management with interdisciplinary team work • Sleep hygiene (AOTA, 2021a; Colletti et al., 2019; Sanjana et al., 2017) • Nutritional management—anti-inflammatory, plant-based, ketogenic, low-carb and low-sugar diets (Field et al., 2022; Schönenberger et al., 2021; Strath et al., 2022)
Fatigue management	• Education about fatigue • Energy conservation techniques • Body mechanics and joint protection • Problem-solving daily scheduling and prioritization of activities using the Spoon Theory • Sleep hygiene (Haynes-Lawrence & West, 2018; Van Heest et al., 2017)
Sleep hygiene	• Relaxation techniques (e.g., progressive muscle relaxation, guided imagery), gentle stretching, yoga, and meditation • Health education • Sleep hygiene education • Sleep diary or log and review • Nutrition and exercise • Education on symptom management • Increased social interaction • Individual and group problem solving, computerized training, didactic class sessions (AOTA, 2021b; Colletti et al., 2019; Fields & Smallfield, 2022; Smallfield & Lucas Molitor, 2018; Van Heest et al., 2017)

(Continued)

TABLE 2.1. Key Habilitative Services to Improve QoL and Engagement in Occupation *(Cont.)*

Theme	Examples

Trauma processing and building resiliency	• Coping skills training
	• Self-awareness and self-esteem
	• Mindfulness
	• Education on trauma triggers and warning signs; developmental issues related to early childhood trauma
	• Symptom stabilization strategies
	• Relaxation techniques
	• Sensory modulation:
	  ○ Therapeutic use of self to connect, assess, and monitor triggers and early warning signs with sensorimotor activities and strategies, grade and adapt
	  ○ Sensory modalities (neurofeedback, sound therapy, weighted items, emotional freedom technique, BAL-A-Vis-X, brushing and tapping with joint compression, Brain Gym, clinical aroma therapy, animal-assisted therapy)
	  ○ Sensory diet
	  ○ Environmental modifications and caregiver involvement (sensory kits and items, sensory spaces, sensory room, sensory cart, personal space, exercise equipment, pet therapy, aromatherapy, areas to walk or hike, movement-based video games, swings and rocking chairs, therapy balls, yoga tools and mats, tactile manipulatives, bean bags, musical instruments, creative crafts and outlets [Champagne, 2019; Kajeepeta et al., 2015; Thoits, 2010])

(Continued)

TABLE 2.1. Key Habilitative Services to Improve QoL and Engagement in Occupation *(Cont.)*

Theme	Examples

Participation in meaningful activities	• Adaptive equipment and compensatory strategies
	  ○ Activity analysis
	  ○ Development of and training in new techniques to maintain participation
	• Using self-management strategies to manage the impact of disease
	• Involvement of caregiver in all aspects of ADL performance (Smallfield et al., 2021)

Note. ADL = activities of daily living; AOTA = American Occupational Therapy Association; BMI = body mass index; COPD = chronic obstructive pulmonary disease; IADLs = instrumental activities of daily living; QoL = quality of life.

Chronic pain management applies to many people with chronic disease, and there is ample evidence for a variety of techniques that have been effective, including mind–body techniques such as relaxation, mindfulness, and self-expression or advocacy; education and acquisition of performance skills related to body mechanics, joint protection, and ergonomics; massage and supports for positioning; adaptations to self-care techniques; and interdisciplinary work for medication management (AOTA, 2021b; Colletti et al., 2019). A unique technique incorporating self-myofascial release, the Melt Method, has evidence for its effectiveness, particularly with low back pain (Hitzman, 2016; Sanjana et al., 2017). There are increasing levels of evidence for the impact of diet on pain, supporting that low amounts of carbohydrates and sugars and avoidance of processed foods result in lower pain levels (Field et al., 2022; Schönenberger et al., 2021; Strath et al., 2022).

Fatigue management includes many techniques similar to those mentioned, but it emphasizes the need to prioritize daily activities, which requires problem solving with support (Haynes-Lawrence & West, 2018; Van Heest et al., 2017). An informal and easy-to-follow energy conservation technique that prioritizes daily activities, called the ***Spoon Theory***, seems to have potential to assist with such prioritization

(Haynes-Lawrence & West, 2018). ***Sleep hygiene*** is significant because it is mentioned in almost every other self-management strategy. Education related to all aspects of sleep is beneficial, as are logging and journaling. Monitoring and increasing daily physical and social activity seem beneficial as well. Finally, trauma processing and building resiliency with sensory modulation is important in dealing with the impact of trauma that may be a primary causative factor of the disease or secondary to it. ***Trauma processing*** involves psychosocial expression, movement activity, and sensory modulation (Champagne, 2019; Kajeepeta et al., 2015; Thoits, 2010). Sensory processing is, interestingly, affected by age and disease, so it needs to be reassessed with grading and adaptation as clients age and disease progresses. Caregivers may be experiencing a decline in health and well-being as a result of their role, so it is important to screen them regularly for the potential need for self-management strategies and make referrals through primary care for occupational therapy services as needed.

Participation in meaningful activity

Participation in ADLs and IADLs is crucial to QoL and also leads to lower health care costs and chance of mortality. This participation has been found to be important to physical, mental, and social well-being (Smallfield et al., 2021). Occupational therapy practitioners have the skills to evaluate current success in participation, analyze demands of the activity, and create adaptations for continued participation despite a decline in client factors or performance skills. Adaptations or compensations may be made through adaptive equipment, compensatory techniques, changes in the environment or context, or establishment of habits and routines. Understanding one's perception of illness is important to successful participation. Shi and Hu (2020) found a positive relationship between one's perception of illness severity and decreased engagement in ADLs, IADLs, role fulfillment, and social activities. Addressing perception through self-management strategies may be a prerequisite to participation goals. Careful involvement of caregivers providing support is imperative to the success of the adaptation.

Other occupational involvement is important as well. As discussed, involvement in social participation has been shown to be very important to QoL (Figure 2.3). Particularly to those who are in terminal care, "occupations specific to the end of life, such as prioritizing

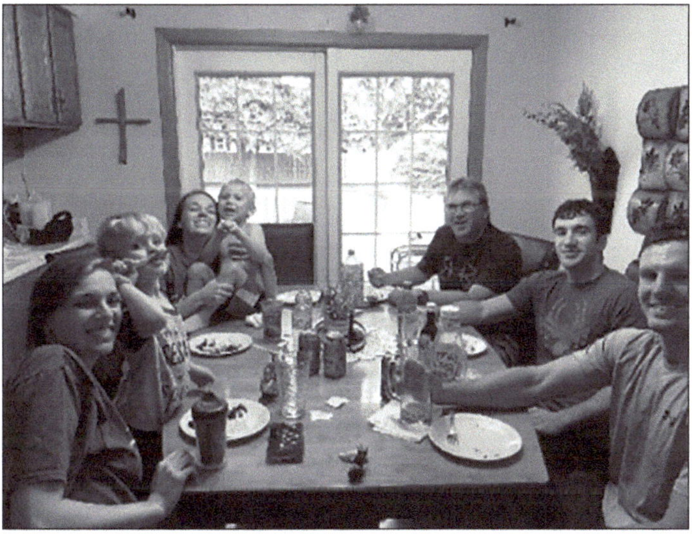

Figure 2.3 Participation in social-based occupations enhances QoL and health.

Source. A. Best. Used with permission.

relationships, reworking life to accommodate illness, engaging in legacy building and life review, finding closure, putting affairs in order, and making final arrangements" (Chow & Pickens, 2020, p. 6) are important and should be included in participation goals for clients and their caregivers.

Road Map for Addressing Chronic Conditions

On the basis of a systematic review of the literature and moderate to strong strength of evidence, Fields and Smallfield (2022) used ***decision-making algorithms*** for determining needs relevant to occupational therapy practice for those with chronic conditions based on a systematic review of the literature and use of moderate to strong evidence. Figure 2.4 shows one such algorithm related to fatigue management.

Similar to their decision algorithms, use of an ***occupational therapy road map*** with those who have chronic disease summarizes the opportunities for meeting needs related to QoL through maintenance programs

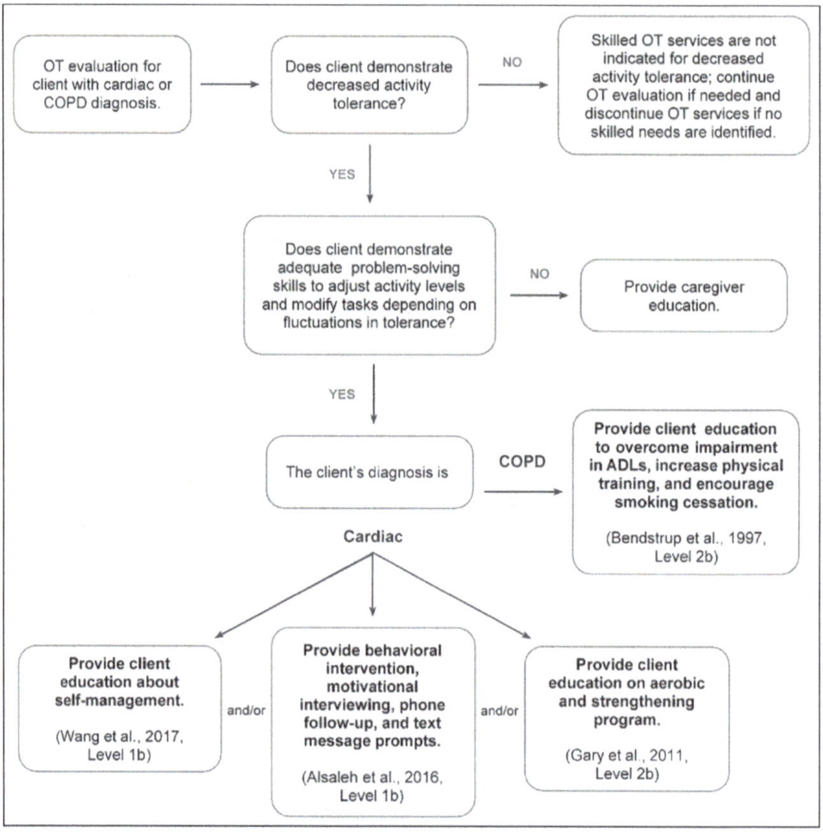

Figure 2.4 Decision-making algorithm for fatigue management.

Note. ADLs = activities of daily living; COPD = chronic obstructive pulmonary disease; OT = occupational therapy.

Source. From "Occupational Therapy Practice Guidelines for Adults With Chronic Conditions," by B. Fields and S. Smallfield, 2022, *American Journal of Occupational Therapy, 76*, p. 16. Copyright © 2022 by the American Occupational Therapy Association.

with specific strategies related to therapeutic use of self, adaptations to environments or contexts to enhance social connections, and habilitation of self-management and participation strategies; care of the caregiver; and involvement in occupational therapy in primary care (see Figure 2.5). Case Examples 2.1 and 2.2 describe use of road maps in occupational therapy practice.

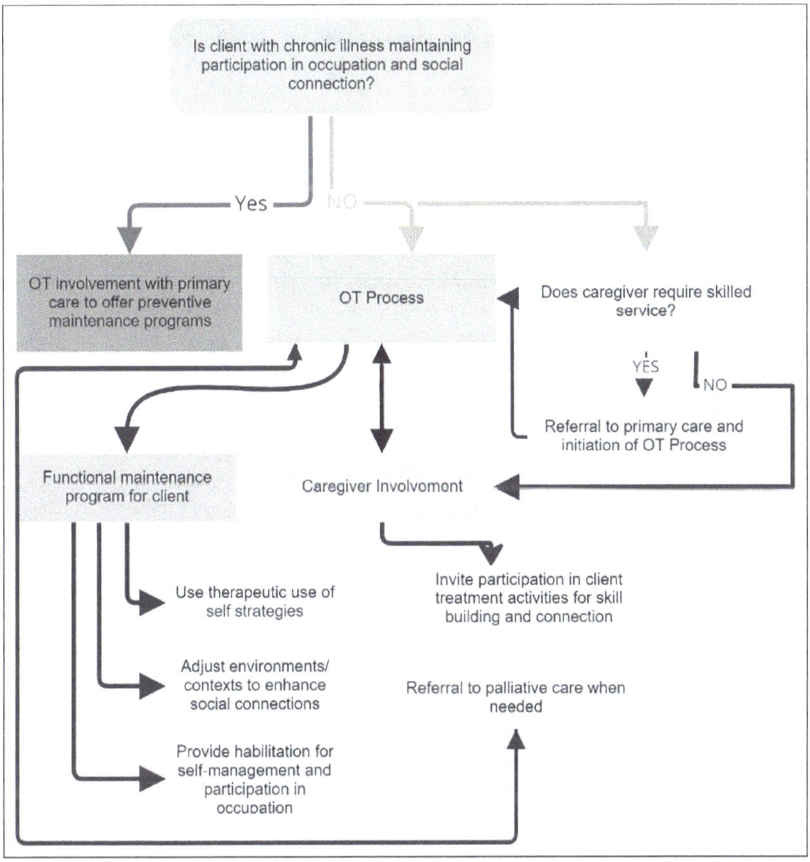

Figure 2.5 Road map for occupational therapy work with people who are chronically ill.

Note. OT = occupational therapy.

Summary

Although occupational therapy practitioners are currently addressing the needs of chronically ill people, opportunities exist to meet needs related to QoL with referral to palliative care when the patient requires "alleviation of suffering and the treatment of physical, psychosocial, and spiritual challenges associated with the illness" (Kurian et al., 2021, p. 1). With chronic illness, there may come a point at which self-management techniques via maintenance programs are not adequate to manage the

CASE EXAMPLE 2.1. MAUREKA: MULTIPLE SCLEROSIS

Maureka is a 65-year-old Black woman who was diagnosed with multiple sclerosis 20 years ago. She had previously been diagnosed with schizophrenia at age 30. She has lived in a skilled nursing facility much of the past 10 years with intermittent attempts to live at home with her children or her mother and sister. She has five children, three of whom have struggled with mental health issues and two of whom have had repetitive issues with law enforcement. She uses a wheelchair but through a functional maintenance program with therapy has had intermittent success with toileting, which has enabled her home visits; however, she is unable to maintain this ability and thus experiences social isolation from her family. When she recently learned of her youngest child's life sentence to prison, she had a significant mental break and a decline in all activity participation. She was referred to occupational therapy, and the occupational therapy evaluation revealed that she had a very strong need for social connection with her family, decreased strength and mobility, and no support from caregivers for toileting because of her current physical status. Occupational therapy intervention involved the following strategies:

- therapeutic use of self, with a focus on empathy and encouragement to facilitate the client's involvement in a self-management physical activity program to increase her activity tolerance
- provision of trauma-informed care and encouragement of trauma processing and sensory modulation related to recently learning of her son's imprisonment
- habilitation of compensatory strategies and adaptive equipment for mobility and toileting skills
- analysis of environment and context with home evaluation and provision of necessary equipment for home visits and set up in room for increased participation in mobility
- active and repetitive touchpoints with caregivers
    - The turnover rate for nurse aides at this facility is high, so the occupational therapy department devised a plan for frequent touchpoints to build relationships with these important caregivers.
        - Share break times with the aides at least once a week, offering carry-in style sharing of meals; use DEI and GLUE (*g*ather, *l*isten, *u*nify, *e*mpower and *e*xecute) leadership techniques to truly connect with these caregivers.
        - During client ADL sessions, set up a long-term maintenance program for clients with chronic illness so they can have ongoing touchpoints with the aides assisting them at least monthly to assess the aides' needs for support to maximize client participation.

(Continued)

CASE EXAMPLE 2.1. MAUREKA: MULTIPLE SCLEROSIS *(Cont.)*

- Family members have difficulty connecting with Maureka and providing the appropriate level of support and are experiencing their own trauma, so the occupational therapist invited them to weekly therapy sessions to allow them to participate in the trauma processing and sensory modulation self-management activities with Maureka in addition to the habilitation of new toileting techniques. The occupational therapist screened them for potential need of occupational therapy services and made a referral for Maureka's sister through her primary care team.

The benefit of the functional maintenance program was the ability to have touchpoint connection for reassessment. At these touchpoints, the occupational therapy practitioner will need to analyze Maureka's level of suffering due to the chronicity of her diseases and facilitate a referral to palliative care when it is warranted.

Note. Case information provided by A. Heffner.

CASE EXAMPLE 2.2. CORISA: CAREGIVER OF A PATIENT WITH CYSTIC FIBROSIS

Corisa is a 42-year-old White woman who is the caregiver for her 17-year-old daughter who has cystic fibrosis (CF). She is married, and her husband has been active as a father but relies on Corisa for caregiving duties for their daughter related to her diagnosis (see Figure 2.6). Corisa is an occupational therapist, so she is familiar with medical culture. She decreased her work schedule to an as-needed basis so that she could work around her caregiver duties. This puts a burden on the family's finances, so she felt responsible for managing them.

After her daughter's initial diagnosis, Corisa experienced a bout of depression that lasted approximately 5 years. She was treated by her primary care physician with medication and experienced significant weight gain during this time. She began experiencing additional symptoms of excessive fatigue and pain that began to affect her caregiving ability, so she sought holistic medical treatment and was diagnosed with "adrenal fatigue" and a gluten intolerance. She altered her diet and lost weight, she used fatigue and chronic pain management strategies that she knew about because of her occupational therapy background, and she was

(Continued)

CASE EXAMPLE 2.2. CORISA: CAREGIVER OF A PATIENT WITH CYSTIC FIBROSIS *(Cont.)*

able to create a life balance that allowed part-time work, active participation in the local CF chapter, and care for her daughter, including exploring and getting her medication that has delayed the progression of the disease.

In addition to her caregiver duties, which have expanded beyond her daughter to the family, she now uses self-management, including diet, sleep hygiene, and chronic fatigue and pain management. She has secured a more permanent job, which allows her flexibility and use of her strategies more consistently than her previous as-needed work. She assisted her daughter with a career plan and recently enjoyed observing her daughter's first romantic relationship blossom. She would benefit from occupational therapy services to assess her need for additional self-management habilitation, including trauma processing and sensory modulation as she continues with her caregiving duties; she is receptive to and appreciative of these services to help her and her daughter participate in life to the fullest. A referral through her primary care team seems appropriate to ensure her QoL as a caregiver.

Note. Case information contributed by C. Ramsey.

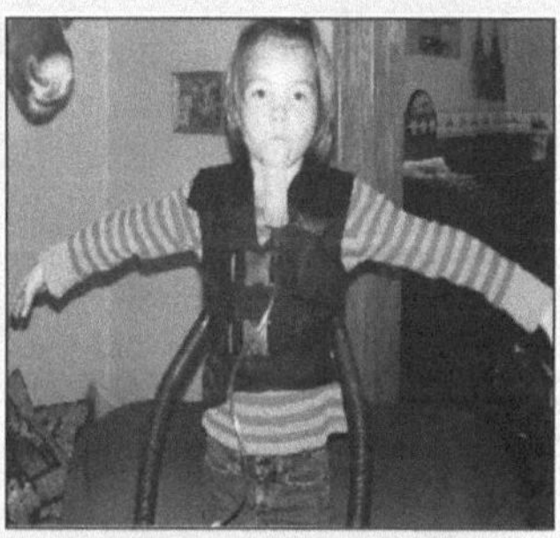

(A)

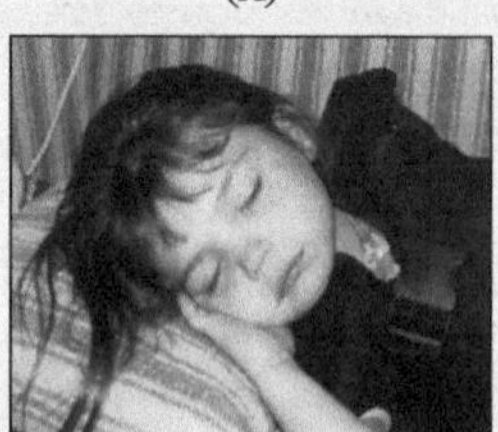

(B)

Figure 2.6 Treatment intervention requiring caregiver application and supervision, including the application of a medical device (A) and providing comfort for rest (B).

suffering experienced. Referral to palliative care can and should happen at any point during the maintenance program when warranted.

Ann B. Best, MHS, OTR/L, is the Assistant Dean of Health Sciences and Public Service at Rhodes State College in Lima, Ohio. She served as the Chair of the Occupational Therapy Assistant Program for 15 years.

REFERENCES

Alsaleh, E., Windle, R., & Blake, H. (2016). Behavioural intervention to increase physical activity in adults with coronary heart disease in Jordan. *BMC Public Health, 16,* 643. https://doi.org/10.1186/s12889-016-3313-5

American Occupational Therapy Association. (2017). Vision 2025. *American Journal of Occupational Therapy, 71,* 7103420010. https://doi.org/10.5014/ajot.2017.713002

American Occupational Therapy Association. (2019). *2019 Salary and Workforce Survey*. AOTA Press.

American Occupational Therapy Association. (2020a). *AOTA's guide to addressing the impact of racial discrimination, stigma, and implicit bias on provision of services.* https://www.aota.org/-/media/corporate/files/practice/dei/addressing-guide-racial-discrimination.pdf

American Occupational Therapy Association. (2020b). Occupational therapy practice framework: Domain and process (4th ed.). *American Journal of Occupational Therapy, 74*(Suppl. 2), 7412410010. https://doi. org/10.5014/ajot.2020.74S2001

American Occupational Therapy Association. (2020c). Occupational therapy's commitment to diversity, equity, and inclusion. *American Journal of Occupational Therapy, 74*(Suppl. 3), 7413410030. https://doi.org/10.5014/ajot.2020.74S3002

American Occupational Therapy Association. (2020d). Role of occupational therapy in primary care. *American Journal of Occupational Therapy, 74*(Suppl. 3), 7413410040. https://doi.org/10.5014/ajot.2020.74S3001

American Occupational Therapy Association (2021a). *AOTA strategic framework.* https://www.aota.org/-/media/corporate/files/aboutaota/2021-aota-strategic-framework.pdf

American Occupational Therapy Association. (2021b). Role of occupational therapy in pain management. *American Journal of Occupational Therapy, 75*(Suppl. 3), 7513410010. https://doi.org/10.5014/ajot.2021.75S3001

American Occupational Therapy Association, American Physical Therapy Association, & American Speech-Language-Hearing Associations. (2021). *Joint habilitation/rehabilitation benefit coverage statement: Guide to assessing adequacy of benefits.* https://www.aota.org/advocacy/issues/health-care-reform/-/media/748073da882f45db993921b3a2aabe1b.ashx

Apostol, C., Cranwell, K., & Hitch, D. (2021). Evaluating a multidimensional strategy to improve the professional self-care of occupational therapists working with people with life limiting illness. *BMC Palliative Care, 20,* 2. https://doi.org/10.1186/s12904-020-00695-x

Baxter, M. F., Newman, R., Longpré, S. M., & Polo, K. M. (2017). Occupational therapy's role in cancer survivorship as a chronic condition. *American Journal of Occupational Therapy, 71,* 7103090010. https://doi.org/10.5014/ajot.2017.713001

Bendstrup, K. E., Ingemann Jensen, J., Holm, S., & Bengtsson, B. (1997). Outpatient rehabilitation improves activities of daily living, quality of life and exercise tolerance in chronic obstructive pulmonary disease. *European Respiratory Journal, 10,* 2801–2806. https://doi.org/10.1183/09031936.97.10122801

Bodenheimer, T., & Sinsky, C. (2014). From Triple to Quadruple Aim: Care of the patient requires care of the provider. *Annals of Family Medicine, 12,* 573–576. https://doi.org/10.1370/afm.1713

Brown, B. (2013). *Brené Brown on empathy* [Video]. RSA Short Video. https://www.thersa.org/video/shorts/2013/12/brene-brown-on-empathy

Carmassi, C., Foghi, C., Dell'Oste, V., Bertelloni, C. A., Fiorillo, A., & Dell'Osso, L. (2020). Risk and protective factors for PTSD in caregivers of adult patients with severe medical illnesses: A systematic review. *International Journal of Environmental Research and Public Health, 17,* 5888. https://doi.org/10.3390/ijerph17165888

Centers for Disease Control and Prevention. (2021a). *About the CDC-Kaiser ACE study.* https://www.cdc.gov/violenceprevention/aces/about.html

Centers for Disease Control and Prevention. (2021b). *Chronic diseases in America.* https://www.cdc.gov/chronicdisease/resources/infographic/chronic-diseases.htm

Centers for Disease Control and Prevention. (2022a). *About chronic diseases.* https://www.cdc.gov/chronicdisease/about/index.htm

Centers for Disease Control and Prevention. (2022b). *What is health equity?* https://www.cdc.gov/nchhstp/healthequity/index.html#:~:text=Health%20equity%20is%20the%20state,their%20highest%20level%20of%20health

Centers for Medicare & Medicaid Services. (2021a). *Frequently asked questions (FAQs) regarding Jimmo Settlement Agreement.* https://www.cms.gov/Center/Special-Topic/Jimmo-Settlement/FAQs

Centers for Medicare & Medicaid Services. (2021b). *Jimmo Settlement.* https://www.cms.gov/Center/Special-Topic/Jimmo-Center

Centers for Medicare & Medicaid Services. (2022). Chapter 15—Covered medical and other health services. In *Medicare benefit policy manual* (Revision 11399). https://www.cms.gov/Regulations-and-Guidance/Guidance/Manuals/Downloads/bp102c15.pdf

Champagne, T. (2019). *Sensory modulation and trauma informed care: An introduction* [Continuing education course]. Making Connections: University of Findlay's Occupational Therapy Continuing Education Series, Findlay, Ohio, United States.

Chapman, G. D. (2010). *The five love languages*. Walker Large Print.

Chow, J. K., & Pickens, N. D. (2020). Measuring the efficacy of occupational therapy in end-of-life care: A scoping review. *American Journal of Occupational Therapy, 74,* 7401205020. https://doi.org/10.5014/ajot.2020.033340

Cole, M. B. (2018). *Group dynamics in occupational therapy* (5th ed.). Slack.

Colletti, M., Levine, D., Heath, G. W., Choo, J., Jones, T., & Mackiewicz, T. (2019). Breaking the pain cycle: A comprehensive multidisciplinary approach to chronic pain management. *American Journal of Occupational Therapy, 73*(4, Suppl. 1), 7311520413. https://doi.org/10.5014/ajot.2019.73S1-PO3030

DeAngelis, T. (2019). The legacy of trauma: An emerging line of research is exploring how historical and cultural traumas affect survivors' children for generations to come. *Monitor on Psychology, 50*(2), 36. https://www.apa.org/monitor/2019/02/legacy-trauma

Early, M. B. (2017). *Mental health concept and techniques for the occupational therapy assistant* (5th ed.). Lippincott Williams & Wilkins.

Fan, C. W., Hazlett, J. N., & Taylor, R. R. (2022). Brief report—Perceiving therapeutic communication: Client–therapist discrepancies. *American Journal of Occupational Therapy, 76,* 7603345010. https://doi.org/10.5014/ajot.2022.047670

Fan, C. W., & Taylor, R. (2018). Correlation between therapeutic use of self and clients' participation in rehabilitation. *American Journal of Occupational Therapy, 72*(4, Suppl. 1), 7211500036. https://doi.org/10.5014/ajot.2018.72S1-PO5001

Fette, C., Lambdin-Pattavina, C., & Weaver, L. (2019). Understanding and applying trauma-informed approaches across occupational therapy settings. *OT Practice, 24*(5), CE1–CE9. https://www.aota.org/-/media/corporate/files/publications/ce-articles/ce-article-may-2019-trauma.pdf

Field, R., Pourkazemi, F., & Rooney, K. (2022). Effects of a low-carbohydrate ketogenic diet on reported pain, blood biomarkers and quality of life in patients with chronic pain: A pilot randomized clinical trial. *Pain Medicine, 23,* 326–338. https://doi.org/10.1093/pm/pnab278

Fields, B., & Smallfield, S. (2022). Occupational therapy practice guidelines for adults with chronic conditions. *American Journal of Occupational Therapy, 76,* 7602397010. https://doi.org/10.5014/ajot.2022/762001

Gary, R. A., Cress, M. E., Higgins, M. K., Smith, A. L., & Dunbar, S. B. (2011). Combined aerobic and resistance exercise program improves task performance in patients with heart failure. *Archives of Physical Medicine and Rehabilitation, 92,* 1371–1381. https://doi.org/10.1016/j.apmr.2011.02.022

Grossman, S., Cooper, Z., Buxton, H., Hendrickson, S., Lewis-O'Connor, A., Stevens, J., . . . Bonne, S. (2021). Trauma-informed care: Recognizing and resisting re-traumatization in health care. *Trauma, Surgery and Acute Care Open, 6*(1), e000815. https://doi.org/10.1136/tsaco-2021-000815

Harding, K. (2019). *The rabbit effect: Live longer, happier, and healthier with the groundbreaking science of kindness.* Simon & Schuster.

Haynes-Lawrence, D., & West, A. R. (2018). Managing fatigue in parents with multiple sclerosis. *Journal of Child and Family Studies, 27,* 1640–1649. https://link.springer.com/article/10.1007/s10826-017-1007-y

Heinemann, A. W., Feuerstein, M., Frontera, W. R., Gard, S. A., Kaminsky, L. A., Negrini, S., Richards, L. G., & Vallée, C. (2020). Rehabilitation is a global health priority. *Archives of Physical Medicine and Rehabilitation, 101,* 728–729. https://doi.org/10.1016/j.apmr.2019.08.468

Hitzman, S. (2016). *The Melt Method.* HarperCollins.

Institute for Healthcare Improvement. (2022). *Triple Aim—The best care for the whole population at the lowest cost.* http://www.ihi.org/Engage/Initiative/TripleAim/Pages/default.aspx

Kajeepeta, S., Gelaye, B., Jackson, C. L., & Williams, M. A. (2015). Adverse childhood experiences are associated with adult sleep disorders: A systematic review. *Sleep Medicine, 16,* 320–330. https://doi.org/10.1016/j.sleep.2014.12.013

Kelly, A. P. (2022). *GLUE: A leadership development strategy to bond and unite.* Trilogy Christian Publishing.

Kulig, J. C., Edge, D. S., Townshend, I., Lightfoot, N., & Reimer, W. (2013). Community resiliency: Emerging theoretical insights. *Journal of Community Psychology, 41,* 758–775. https://doi.org/10.1002/jcop.21569

Kurian, S., Kramer, J. M., O'Rourke, B. O., Rocco, C., & Newman, R. (2021). Meaning making while living with life-threatening illness. *OT Practice.* https://www.aota.org/publications/ot-practice/ot-practice-issues/2021/meaning-making-palliative-care

Lehrner, A., & Yehuda, R. (2018). Cultural trauma and epigenetic inheritance. *Development and Psychopathology, 30,* 1763–1777. https://doi.org/10.1017/S0954579418001153

Leland, N. E., Fogelberg, D. J., Halle, A. D., & Mroz, T. M. (2017). Occupational therapy and management of multiple chronic conditions in the context of health care reform. *American Journal of Occupational Therapy, 71,* 7101090010. https://doi.org/10.5014/ajot.2017.711001

Martino, J., Pegg, J., & Frates, E. P. (2015). The connection prescription: Using the power of social interactions and the deep desire for connectedness to empower health and wellness. *American Journal of Lifestyle Medicine, 11,* 466–475. https://doi.org/10.1177/1559827615608788

Murphy, A. D., Griffith, V. M., Berkeridge, T., Mroz, T. M., & Jirikowic, T. L. (2017). Health Policy Perspectives—Primary care for underserved populations: Navigating policy to incorporate occupational therapy into federally qualified health centers. *American Journal of Occupational Therapy, 71,* 7102090010. https://doi.org/10.5014/ajot.2017.712001

Novak, L., & Jewell, V. (2020). The effect of education on knowledge and perceptions of nursing staff regarding functional maintenance programs: A pilot study. *American Journal of Occupational Therapy, 74*(4, Suppl. 1), 7411505253. https://doi.org/10.5014/ajot.2020.74S1-PO9608

Nundy, S., Cooper, L. A., & Mate, K. S. (2022). The quintuple aim for health care improvement: A new imperative to advance health equity. *JAMA, 327,* 521–522. https://doi.org/10.1001/jama.2021.25181

O'Brien, M. (2019, April 8). *How to have more empathy: Learn the four attributes of empathy from Brené Brown.* Mrs. Mindfulness. https://mrsmindfulness.com/four-attributes-of-empathy-brene-brown/

Patient Protection and Affordable Care Act, Pub. L. 111-148, 42 U.S.C. §§ 18001–18121 (2010).

Perez, G. K., Haime, V., Jackson, V., Chittenden, E., Mehta, D. H., & Park, E. R. (2015). Promoting resiliency among palliative care clinicians: Stressors, coping strategies, and training needs. *Journal of Palliative Medicine, 18,* 332–337. https://doi.org/10.1089/jpm.2014.0221

Rafeedie, S., Metzler, C., & Lamb, A. J. (2018). Health policy perspectives—Opportunities for occupational therapy to serve as a catalyst for culture change in nursing facilities. *American Journal of Occupational Therapy, 72,* 7204090010. https://pubmed.ncbi.nlm.nih.gov/29953823/

Rouch, S. A., Klinedinst, T. C., White, J. S., & Leland, N. E. (2022). Exploring occupational therapists' experiences in U.S. primary care settings: A qualitative study. *American Journal of Occupational Therapy, 76,* 7601180010. https://doi.org/10.5014/ajot.2022.049001

Sanjana, F., Chaudhry, H., & Findley, T. (2017). Effect of MELT method on thoracolumbar connective tissue: The full study. *Journal of Bodywork and Movement Therapies, 21,* 179–185. https://doi.org/10.1016/j.jbmt.2016.05.010

Schönenberger, K. A., Schüpfer, A.-C., Gloy, V. L., Hasler, P., Stanga, Z., Kaegi-Braun, N., & Reber, E. (2021). Effect of anti-inflammatory diets on pain in rheumatoid arthritis: A systematic review and meta-analysis. *Nutrients, 13*(12), 4221. https://doi.org/10.3390/nu13124221

Schoultz, E. D. (2021). Caregivers' experiences of unmet needs for emotional intimacy while caring for chronically ill spouses (Publication No. 28153369) [Doctoral dissertation, Capella University, Minneapolis, MN].

Seymour, A. (2012). The use of self in occupational therapy. In G. Boniface & A. Seymour (Eds.), *Using occupational therapy in practice* (pp. 49–59). Blackwell. https://doi.org/10.1002/9781118709634.ch5

Shi, M. H., & Mu, H. (2020). Do people's beliefs about their illness affect their engagement in daily routine activities? *American Journal of*

Occupational Therapy, 74(4, Suppl. 1), 7411505172. https://doi.org/10.5014/ajot.2020.74S1-PO5723

Smallfield, S., & Lucas Molitor, W. (2018). Occupational therapy interventions addressing sleep for community-dwelling older adults: A systematic review. *American Journal of Occupational Therapy, 72,* 7204190030. https://doi.org/10.5014/ajot.2018.031211

Smallfield, S., Fang, L., & Kyler, D. (2021). Self-management interventions to improve activities of daily living and rest and sleep for adults with chronic conditions: A systematic review. *American Journal of Occupational Therapy, 75,* 7504190010. https://doi.org/10.5014/ajot.2021.046946

Soper, K. (2022). Reducing burnout and promoting professional development in the palliative care service. *Journal of Hospice and Palliative Nursing, 24,* 181–185. https://doi-org.proxy.ohiolink.edu:9100/10.1097/NJH.0000000000000847

Stern, B. Z. (2019). Expanding self-management support from chronic to acute care: Implications for value. *American Journal of Occupational Therapy, 73,* 7303347010. https://doi.org/10.5014/ajot.2019.030007

Strath, L. J., Brooks, M. S., Sorge, R. E., & Judd, S. E. (2022). Relationship between diet and relative risk of pain in a cross-sectional analysis of the REGARDS longitudinal study. *Pain Management, 12,* 168–179. https://doi.org/10.2217/pmt-2021-0048

Stuart, C. (2020). Empathy and the student–teacher relationship: How to read behavioural cues. *Teachers Matter, 47,* 10–11.

Taylor, R. R. (2008). *The intentional relationship: Occupational therapy and use of self.* F. A. Davis.

Thoits, P. A. (2010). Stress and health: Major findings and policy implications. *Journal of Health and Social Behavior, 51*(Suppl.), S41–S53. https://doi.org/10.1177/0022146510383499

Van Heest, K. N., Mogush, A., & Mathiowetz, V. G. (2017). Effects of a one-to-one fatigue management course for people with chronic conditions and fatigue. *American Journal of Occupational Therapy, 71,* 7104100020. https://doi.org/10.5014/ajot.2017.023440

Wang, Q., Dong, L., Jian, Z., & Tang, X. (2017). Effectiveness of a PRECEDE-based education intervention on quality of life in elderly patients with chronic heart failure. *BMC Cardiovascular Disorders, 17,* 262. https://doi.org/10.1186/s12872-017-0698-8

Weinstein, E. (1998). Elements of the art of practice in mental health. *American Journal of Occupational Therapy, 52,* 579–585. https://doi.org/10.5014/ajot.52.7.579

Yerxa, E. J. (1992). Some implications of occupational therapy's history for its epistemology, values, and relation to medicine. *American Journal of Occupational Therapy, 46,* 79–83. https://doi.org/10.5014/ajot.46.1.79

3

Palliative Care and Occupational Therapy

CHRISTIAN H. JACOBUS, MD, FACEP, FAAHPM,
and LINDSEY BUDDELMEYER, OTD, MOT, OTR/L

Learning Objectives

After completing this chapter, readers will be able to

- define the core constructs of palliative care,
- describe different service delivery models in the U.S. health care system,
- explain the roles of traditional members of the care team,
- describe pharmacological versus nonpharmacological intervention strategies,
- describe the occupational therapy practitioner's role on the palliative care team, and
- provide case examples to illustrate application of the concepts discussed.

Key Terms and Concepts

chaplains
goals of care
holistic approach
hospice
nurse
nurse practitioner
occupation
palliative care
palliative care physician
palliative medicine
physician
physician assistant
plan of care
social worker
total pain
wrap-around services

According to the Centers for Disease Control and Prevention (CDC), 6 in 10 adults are living with a chronic illness. Moreover, 4 in 10 adults are living with two or more chronic conditions (National Center for Chronic Disease Prevention, 2021). Occupational therapy practitioners are trained providers who routinely work with and treat those facing chronic illness. However, current practice involving the chronic disease community more often occurs from a reactive than a proactive standpoint. Consequently, occupational therapy practitioners are traditionally only called in to address an acute, subacute, or exacerbation type of situation involving the patient. This practice lends itself to a very siloed look at the patient and a limited ability to attend to and address the comorbidities that often accompany chronic illness.

Palliative care is a model of health care that believes in helping patients manage their symptoms to improve their quality of life (QoL). This is done by providing interdisciplinary care and wrap-around services that are tailored and supportive to meet the unique needs of each patient. ***Wrap-around services*** is a term to explain different services addressing different needs and challenges that the patient and family may face. The services "wrap around" and make them feel more supported by providing a proactive approach. In palliative care, an infrastructure supports the workings of the care team to assist patients along the trajectory of their illness and to prevent unnecessary hospitalizations. In lay terms, this model's design affords health care professionals the opportunity to work with patients and their families in an ongoing way. This approach offers those facing chronic illness the ability to feel more supported knowing an additional team of trained professionals is there to assist, provide, and manage their care.

This chapter provides information in relation to the fundamental philosophy and core constructs of palliative care practice and describes the distinct role of occupational therapy practitioners on the palliative care team.

Occupational Therapy and Reframing Our Role in the Medical Community

Occupational therapy practitioners are trained health care professionals who work with patients of all ages and abilities from birth to death.

When patients are facing an incurable condition, practitioners will often be pulled in and out of cases in tandem with the patient's most recent hospitalization or exacerbation. It is within the confines of these already well-established spaces that clinicians begin to identify and speak about recurrent patients as "frequent fliers," or abusers of the emergency department (ED; Coleman et al., 2001). Although this perception of overuse of the ED may be true, is it fair to label medically complex patients in this way? Or is the U.S. health care system inevitably setting these patients up to fail, particularly if they are receiving only formalized care through their attending provider versus interdisciplinary and skilled care services from the time they receive their diagnosis and thereafter as their disease progresses?

A core and founding construct of the occupational therapy profession is the way in which occupations are viewed. The term ***occupation*** stretches well beyond simply a job; it embodies any personalized activity that patients engage in that brings purpose and meaning to their life (American Occupational Therapy Association [AOTA], 2020). Incorporating this viewpoint on occupation into clinical practice, providing therapeutic use of self when interacting and working with others, being patient and caregiver centered and driven, and using theory to guide work with patients are all cornerstones of and contributors to what makes occupational therapy unique and distinctly different from other professions.

Worldwide, occupational therapy practitioners are working with patients diagnosed with various types of chronic illness. In fact, most practitioners will work with people with chronic illness or will encounter those facing the end of life at some point during their career (Maciejewski et al., 2017). However, the model of care used in chronic care is housed in a more traditional rehabilitation setting and space. Naturally, through past practice, the professional and lay communities may only think of occupational therapy practitioners as being present in skilled nursing facilities, hospitals, and clinics that strictly use a rehabilitation model. This thinking affects when and whether a health care provider ever requests occupational therapy services for a patient. Educating both lay and professional communities and reframing when it is appropriate to call occupational therapy into cases and under what models of care they can treat patients will help to promote occupational therapy practitioners' work in palliative medicine.

Traditional Health Care Approaches and Service Delivery Models

Palliative care exists to focus on the comfort and QoL of patients with life-altering medical problems. The word *palliative* comes from the Latin *pallium,* meaning "cloak." This etymology is illustrative in that palliative care seeks to soothe or "cover" distressing symptoms rather than cure the underlying disease. Providers improve QoL by using comfort-oriented medications (e.g., analgesics, anxiolytics, antiemetics, antidepressants) but also by helping patients make informed decisions about potentially burdensome tests or treatments. The palliative care model's focus on comfort contrasts with the traditional health care mindset that emphasizes cure. For example, if an older adult patient feels that she would not want treatment for colon cancer, then it may not make sense to proceed with a screening colonoscopy. If a patient with dementia is in his last few weeks of life and fatigues with activity, then pursuing rehabilitation may not be the best use of his limited resources of time and energy. In short, palliative care asks the question, "Just because we can proceed with an intervention, *should we*?"

Although comfort and cure are often perceived to be dichotomous, they do not have to be mutually exclusive. There is significant overlap where a patient can receive both life-prolonging care and meticulous symptom management. This overlap is the domain of palliative care. As previously mentioned, the idea that good symptom management and prolonging life are at odds is not always accurate. For many diseases, comfort medication used in judicious amounts does not affect life expectancy (Verberkt et al., 2020); for some kinds of cancer, the involvement of a palliative care provider and high-quality symptom management actually prolong life (Sullivan et al., 2019; Temel et al., 2010). Occupational therapy can be a valuable nonpharmacological palliative intervention, offering patients support in pursuing their valued occupations.

A Newer Model to Consider: Palliative Care's Philosophy and Constructs

The Center to Advance Palliative Care (2022) defines *palliative care* as

> specialized medical care for people living with a serious illness . . . focused on providing relief from the symptoms and stress of the illness. The goal is to

> improve QoL for both the patient and the family. Palliative care is provided by a specially-trained team of doctors, nurses and other specialists who work together with a patient's other doctors to provide an extra layer of support.... It is appropriate at any age and at any stage in a serious illness, and it can be provided along with curative treatment. (Center to Advance Palliative Care, 2022, para. 2)

Multiple points in this definition deserve particular attention. Note that palliative care is appropriate for anyone with a serious illness; it is not limited to patients with cancer or with a terminal illness, as is often believed. The goal of palliative care is to relieve suffering and improve QoL, not to cure an illness or prolong life. Palliative care is ideally delivered by a team with a ***holistic approach*** to medical, psychological, and spiritual care (see Table 3.1). Palliative care providers work with a patient's other providers, not as a replacement for them, to better understand a patient's complete medical picture. It can be provided for children and even prenatally. Arguably most important, it can be delivered alongside curative or life-prolonging treatment. Hospice care (a particular type of palliative care discussed in more detail in the next chapter) requires the cessation of aggressive curative treatments, but palliative care in general does not.

Hospice is a special form of palliative care that is reserved for patients who are believed to be in their last 6 months of life and are ready to stop curative treatment for their terminal illness. Although in general palliative care is billed the same way other provider visits are billed, hospice is usually billed under the Medicare Hospice Benefit and comes with a set of specific rules and regulations about how the care is delivered.

HOLISTIC APPROACH

The holistic nature of palliative care warrants further exploration. Physical symptoms such as pain, shortness of breath, nausea, and anxiety are significant contributors to suffering, but social, psychological, and spiritual distress can play equally important roles. This observation of the contribution of nonphysical domains to suffering is the concept of ***total pain,*** an idea advanced by Dame Cicely Saunders, the founder of modern hospice (Clark, 1999; see Figure 3.1). She posited that, for example, when a patient with end-stage cancer reports a pain level of 8 out of 10, only some of that suffering is physical distress. Social factors such as isolation

TABLE 3.1. Palliative Care Core Team Roles

Role	Possible Duties
Physician, nurse practitioner, physician assistant	• Evaluate symptom burden • Directly manage or make recommendations for comfort medications • Discuss goals of care
Social worker	• Assess and treat psychosocial sources of suffering • Advise on financial and insurance issues • Assist with completion of advance directives • Assist with placing a patient in a facility • Make recommendations for and assist in obtaining medical equipment • Assess need and qualification for community resources • May: ∘ Discuss goals of care
Chaplain	• Assess and treat spiritual, existential, and emotional sources of suffering • May: ∘ Assess and treat psychosocial sources of suffering

Nurse	• Perform follow-up visits
	• Take medication history
	• May:
	  ∘ Evaluate symptom burden
	  ∘ Assist with completion of advance directives
	  ∘ Discuss goals of care
	  ∘ Make recommendations for comfort medications
	  ∘ Assess psychosocial and spiritual sources of suffering

from friends, psychological factors such as depression and anxiety, and spiritual factors such as anger at God for their situation are also part of their suffering. To focus only on the physical aspect of suffering is to ignore huge parts of a patient's life that might be causing even more distress than pain is. This focus on the nonphysical aspects of suffering also allows

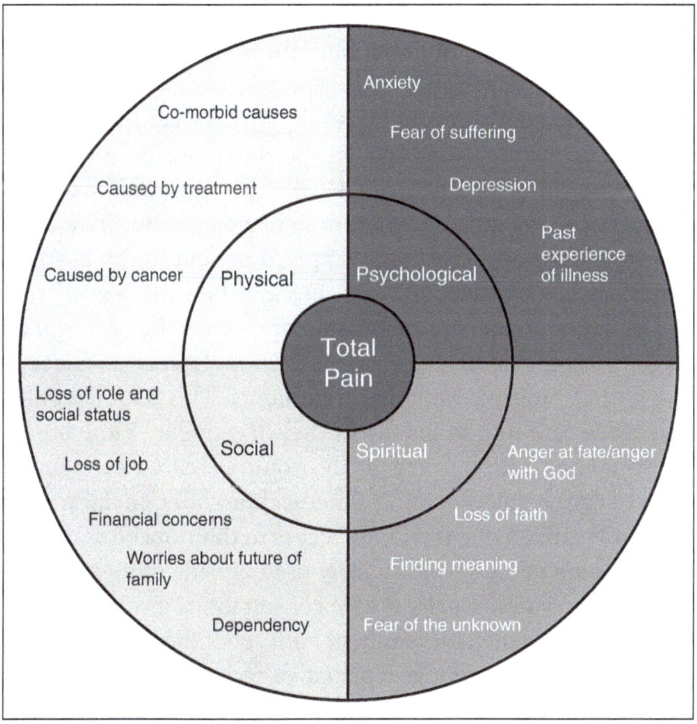

Figure 3.1 Total pain.

Source. Franklin & Lovell (2018). Copyright © 2018 by Springer. Used with permission.

palliative care providers to give social, psychological, and spiritual support to the patient's family and friends.

ACCESS

Palliative care can be accessed in a variety of settings and circumstances: inpatient or outpatient, home (which includes nursing homes or assisted living facilities), or clinic. Larger palliative care teams will have a provider (physician, nurse practitioner, or physician assistant), nurse, social worker, and chaplain, but smaller palliative care services may include only one of those positions. The most common reasons for a palliative care consultation, either inpatient or outpatient, are symptom management and discussion of goals of care. Teams responding to symptom management consultations may make recommendations to the primary team, take over the management of burdensome symptoms, or even take over care as the primary team.

Some larger hospitals have dedicated palliative care units where patients can receive care from specialty-trained nurses and therapists. Patients appropriate for a dedicated palliative care unit would have a primary goal of comfort and symptom management but may not yet be ready or eligible for hospice. For example, a patient in the hospital with cancer that has metastasized to the bones may be getting a 10-treatment course of radiation to palliate that pain. For reasons that are explained in Chapter 4, "Hospice and Occupational Therapy," most hospices cannot cover the cost of multiple radiation treatments. This patient could come to the palliative care unit to finish out their treatment before moving out of the hospital and into hospice. They would be cared for primarily by the palliative care team, including a medical provider, social worker, and chaplain, while still having inpatient access to their oncologist.

The term ***goals of care*** is not widely used outside of medicine and deserves some explanation. Goals-of-care consultations involve detailed conversations with a patient, their family, or both about their current and future medical treatment. For example, a palliative care team may meet with the family of a patient with dementia to discuss the advantages and disadvantages of inserting a feeding tube. The team may meet with an elderly cancer patient who is in the hospital because of the side effects of cytotoxic chemotherapy to discuss whether to continue cancer treatment. These conversations can be long and detailed and may include questions such as

- What is important to you in your life?
- Are you looking for more time to live, more comfort, or both?
- How much suffering are you willing to put up with if it means you can live longer?
- What QoL would be acceptable for you?
- Are the treatments you are currently receiving doing what you want them to?

These conversations can also be held with the family if a patient is unable to converse. For example, consider a patient who has had a severe stroke and has been expressing to his family for months that he is ready to die and would never want to live in a nursing home. To honor his goals, it may be more appropriate to choose hospice than to admit the patient to the hospital for workup, therapy, and placement in a rehabilitation facility. Another example is an elderly patient with advanced dementia who is in the hospital for aspiration pneumonia due to worsening dysphagia. In a discussion of his goals, it comes out that he always told his family that he would not want to be kept alive artificially. Comfort care and pleasure feedings would be more aligned with his goals than insertion of a feeding tube and nothing-by-mouth status.

Outpatient programs are typically structured similarly to inpatient ones but almost always include a provider. They can be based out of a clinic, but, because the target population includes patients with advanced illness and debility, programs that come to patients wherever they are living are common.

Hospice is a special form of palliative care that is only for patients who are close to the end of life and are ready to stop life-prolonging treatment. It is an insurance benefit and an entire system of care that focuses on comfort in the final few months. It includes medical care brought to wherever the patient calls home as well as social, psychological, and spiritual support. It also covers the cost of medical equipment and medications and is discussed in more detail in Chapter 4.

DIAGNOSES

There are no hard-and-fast rules about which diagnoses are appropriate for palliative care. A common misconception is that palliative care is only appropriate for cancer patients, but that is not the case. Any diagnosis that significantly affects a patient's life and sense of well-being is eligible. Common diagnoses are organ failure syndromes such as congestive heart failure, kidney failure, liver failure, and dementia (brain failure). Patients with a diagnosis with an expected decline, such as Huntington's disease, multiple sclerosis, and amyotrophic lateral sclerosis, are also very appropriate for palliative care. Patients with diagnoses that carry a limited prognosis with the risk of a sudden rapid decline (the so-called ticking time bomb), such as a large abdominal aortic aneurysm, cerebral aneurysm, or nonintervenable coronary artery disease, are also eligible.

Palliative care interventions vary widely depending on the disease. A patient with newly diagnosed Huntington's disease may be having minimal physical symptoms but extreme anxiety from the knowledge of their impeding decline and a spiritual crisis because they are questioning why

God has forsaken them. A patient with a spinal cord injury may benefit from counseling about the risk of recurrent pressure injuries from being immobile in bed and from exploring whether they would want to be intubated if they developed pneumonia. A patient with advanced dementia may get frequent urinary tract infections, and the palliative care team may discuss with the patient's decision maker when it might be the right time to not treat the next infection.

EVIDENCE

As one of the newest specialties in medicine, palliative care is still developing an evidence base to support its use. Many studies are observational or underpowered, but their quality improves every year. The data so far indicate that, when palliative care is involved in a patient's care, the patient has better control of both pain and nonpain symptoms (Casarett et al., 2010). It leads to earlier family meetings when a patient is in intensive care, shorter hospital lengths of stay (Braus et al., 2015), and fewer readmissions to the intensive care unit (Gade et al., 2008). Patients, families, and the providers who referred them to palliative care have improved satisfaction (Gade et al., 2008). Health care spending is lower among palliative care patients (Gade et al., 2008; Lustbader et al., 2017; May et al., 2015), as is aggressive care in the weeks and months leading up to death (Jang et al., 2015; Lustbader et al., 2017). Consistent with palliative care's mission of also caring for the families of patients, lower rates of posttraumatic stress disorder and complicated grief are seen among the bereaved (Dionne-Odom et al., 2015). In some cases, prolonged survival of patients is also seen. At first this seems incongruous, given palliative care's emphasis on comfort rather than more time to live, but the hypothesis is that, with meticulous symptom management, a patient can tolerate more cancer treatment and thus live longer (Bakitas et al., 2015; Temel et al., 2010).

Palliative Care Interdisciplinary Team Members

A physician, nurse practitioner, or physician assistant seeing patients solo to address symptoms or goals of care is practicing ***palliative medicine.*** Palliative *care* is provided by a team. The core team members represent the medical, social, psychological, and spiritual domains of suffering. A nurse, nurse practitioner, physician's assistant, or physician could be addressing medical needs. A registered or practical ***nurse*** would be able to have goals-of-care conversations and may have enough experience to make recommendations on symptom management to the referring provider, but they would be unable to prescribe or write orders. A provider such as a ***physician, physician assistant,*** or ***nurse practitioner*** could also directly manage symptoms by prescribing medications or writing inpatient orders.

A ***social worker*** is the team member who most commonly addresses the social and psychological domains, although a chaplain may also be comfortable addressing psychological distress. Working in those domains, the social worker could perform counseling, such as cognitive-behavioral therapy for posttraumatic stress disorder; assisting a patient in applying for Medicaid; or helping to place them in a higher level of care. Depending on their level of medical experience, a social worker or chaplain may also be able to have goals-of-care conversations. ***Chaplains*** address the spiritual side of suffering and, depending on their background, may be able to perform important rituals such as anointing of the sick, weddings, and funerals. They can help with crises of faith, existential distress, and bereavement.

Dating back to 1972, the Institute of Medicine has issued a call to action to provide patients with a team-based approach as a means of improving patient safety and outcomes. In fact, evidence indicates that when interdisciplinary palliative care teams are involved, this approach results in improved outcomes not only for patients but also for caregivers and health systems (Ferrell et al., 2015). "A collaborative interprofessional care team supports high quality and safe care, patient and staff satisfaction and engagement, and organizational efficiency and innovation" (Morley & Cashell, 2017, p. 213). Contemporized palliative care teams require a slight shift in thinking—for example, pulling in an occupational therapy practitioner to work in collaboration with a medical doctor, nurse practitioner, social worker, and chaplain to provide skilled care under a palliative care model. An occupational therapy practitioner brings the distinct value of providing everyday life solutions to help support patients and caregivers in their ability to engage in meaningful and purposeful life activities, feeding into the overall shared belief of palliative medicine that health care is a collaborative and shared experience among the patient and providers and is aimed at improving overall QoL.

Evaluation, Frequency, and Visits

EVALUATION

There is a significant amount of variability in the way palliative care programs staff their teams. Some may use a nurse or a social worker for the initial admission visit. It is common, though, for a provider (a physician, nurse practitioner, or physician assistant) to perform the initial evaluation or intake. These initial visits are often long and comprehensive. This author's (Jacobus) palliative care program schedules 90 minutes for initial visits. This evaluation includes discussion of the patient's current medical issues; a complete symptom inventory; discussion of goals of care, including resuscitation preferences; assessment of psychological, social, and spiritual needs; discussion with the family, referring provider, or both; and the development of a plan. Although other disciplines need to be available, they may not be needed for every patient. The provider typically determines which other disciplines will be required. For example, if a patient is not very religious, then a chaplain visit may be more burdensome than comforting.

PLAN OF CARE

Usually, the ***plan of care*** for a patient will include pharmacological treatment. Depending on the makeup of the team, medications could be prescribed directly or recommended to the referring provider. Medications for pain, shortness of breath, nausea, and anxiety are common. The team may also order or recommend nonpharmacological treatment options. For example, palliative surgery could be recommended for an older patient with dementia and a hip fracture; paracentesis might be ordered for a patient in liver failure; cognitive-behavioral therapy may be appropriate for a veteran with posttraumatic stress disorder; spiritual counseling could assist with a patient's existential distress; and social work could help get a patient with declining functional ability into a facility that can support a higher level of care. Most relevant to the subject of this chapter, physical, occupational, and speech therapy can be ordered to help with strength, balance, coordination, and cognition and can target the support of everyday life activities through interventions and caregiver education.

FOLLOW UP

After a patient's initial visit, the frequency, duration, and thoroughness of subsequent encounters can vary widely between palliative care agencies. A smaller inpatient service may see a patient once to establish goals of care and then not see them again. A larger inpatient service may see patients daily until discharge. A smaller outpatient service may see patients once every 2 to 3 months; a larger program may be able to see patients as often as weekly. Visit frequency is dictated by the abilities of the program and the needs of the patient. Palliative care patients are, by their nature, sick and often getting sicker, so frequent visits or a robust system of telephone follow-ups can help with timely symptom management and earlier referrals into hospice. Telehealth appointments, made much more common during the SARS-CoV-2 virus (COVID-19) pandemic (Baum et al., 2021), are also a way to improve tracking of patients between in-person visits. This author's (Jacobus) program aims for routine visits every 4 to 6 weeks, with more frequent visits or phone calls as symptoms worsen and decline progresses.

Follow-up visits are usually shorter than the initial visit but may still last an hour or longer, particularly when discussing changing goals of care. As a patient's disease progresses, it may be necessary to reexamine their current QoL, the interventions they are currently receiving, and whether those interventions are helping the patient reach their goal. Continuous reassessment of goals can help ensure that patients' needs are being met and that they are referred to hospice at the right time. Follow-up visits are also a good time to assess the efficacy of the current plan, especially symptom management interventions. The Edmonton Symptom Assessment System is a commonly used symptom inventory for palliative care patients (Bruera et al., 1991). It addresses 10 common burdensome symptoms and asks patients to rate each symptom on a scale ranging from 0 to 10, with 0 = *no symptoms at all* and 10 = *severe*. The Palliative Performance Scale (Anderson et al., 1996) and the Karnofsky Performance Scale (Karnofsky et al., 1948) are almost universally used in palliative care programs to track patients' overall level of function and to track decline.

CARE COORDINATION

Coordination of care is a significant part of palliative care's mission. It is common for a patient to have multiple specialists, in addition to their primary care provider, addressing the same issue from different perspectives. For example, a patient with a brain tumor might have a neurosurgeon, neurologist, medical oncologist, and radiation oncologist all contributing to their care, weighing in on disease progression or treatment efficacy, and prescribing medications. Although this is a strength of interdisciplinary care, in a situation such as that it is easy for a patient to hear conflicting information or receive multiple prescriptions for the same symptom. With its holistic philosophy and emphasis on communicating with the patient, palliative care is well suited to help coordinate care. It is vital to note, though, that palliative care does not replace a patient's team of providers but instead acts as a liaison between different specialties and the patient.

Billing

It is difficult for a palliative care program to make a profit on its own. With a significant amount of unbillable travel time and a patient population who often have need for phone time between visits, actual billable hours can be low. Social work interventions may be billable if the provider is independently licensed, but only if the time is spent doing counseling. Spiritual care visits are never billable. Physical, occupational, and speech therapy services are billable and may help with a program's financial viability if the program provides them, rather than referring out to another institution. The real financial value of a palliative care program comes from its impact on an associated hospice and hospital system. Palliative care has been shown to improve patient experience scores, 30-day readmission rates, hospital mortality, and cost per Medicare beneficiary, all of which is publicly available information (Stevens & Bowman, 2020); thus, it can have a serious impact on a hospital system's bottom line. For an associated hospice program, having a palliative care service means earlier hospice enrollment and more billable days (Scheffey et al., 2014).

Summary

Palliative care is a medical specialty that focuses on comfort and QoL (see Case Examples 3.1–3.3). Medical providers manage distressing symptoms and help patients consider the value and detriments of their current medical care and any that might be proposed by their medical team. Occupational therapy, with its focus on activities that bring meaning and purpose to a patient's life, is well suited to be part of a palliative treatment plan. Palliative care aims to minimize suffering by addressing not only the physical dimensions of distress, but also the spiritual, social, and psychological domains. It can be delivered in an inpatient or outpatient setting by a health care provider, nurse, social worker, chaplain, or any combination of these roles. As seen in the case examples, the addition of an occupational therapy practitioner to the team adds valuable perspective and expertise to the holistic care of complex patients.

CASE EXAMPLE 3.1. JOHN: ALZHEIMER'S DISEASE AND PALLIATIVE CARE

John is an 82-year-old man with moderate to severe Alzheimer's disease, referred by his neurologist to the Skills2Care program. The Skills2Care program is embedded in the palliative care service of a local home health and hospice agency. He was seen at home by the occupational therapist, who noted a recent increase in difficulty with daily caregiving because of his progressive disease. He scored 9 out of 30 on the Montreal Cognitive Assessment, indicating severe impairment (Nasreddine et al., 2005). He had difficulty with bathing and dressing and had fatigue and sleepiness throughout the day. He had disrupted sleep at night and periods of incontinence of bowel and bladder. He was unable to safely manage his own medications. His gait was also noted to be unsteady, increasing his risk for falls.

John's wife, Betty, who was his primary caregiver, was having increasing trouble caring for him and meeting his needs. She had chronic leukemia and was slowly getting weaker as well. She had limited knowledge of Alzheimer's disease, and so she did not know what to expect as his disease progressed. She was experiencing social isolation as a result of increased caregiving. In addition, their children, who lived out of town, did not see his decline as acutely as she did and were unaware

(Continued)

CASE EXAMPLE 3.1. JOHN: ALZHEIMER'S DISEASE AND PALLIATIVE CARE *(Cont.)*

of her struggles to care for him. Her practice for administering medications was to keep his pill bottles out on the table and verbally remind him when it was time to take them. This resulted in confusion on his part, frustration on both of their parts, and many missed doses of medication. The occupational therapist recommended keeping the pill bottles out of sight, using a medication organizer or dispenser, physically handing him the pills and water, and assisting him with taking the pills one at a time.

The occupational therapist noted that bathing was an area in which their current practice was unsafe as well. John was showering unassisted, was likely not cleaning appropriately, and was at risk for falls. She instructed them in safe procedures for shower transfers, the sequence of steps to ensure proper hygiene, and obtaining necessary equipment.

John's family had questions about goals of care. He had been having urinary hesitancy and a rising prostate-specific antigen level, and Urology was recommending a prostate biopsy. His family was not sure they wanted to proceed with that test. Betty requested that he be seen by the ***palliative care physician*** to further discuss his family's goals for him.

The physician met with John and his family to do a medical assessment and discuss goals. His family told the physician that family is one of John's main priorities. He also really enjoyed getting out to breakfast with other retirees from his former company but had been unable to do so lately. They felt that his current QoL was acceptable and wanted him to be able to live longer as long as he could keep a reasonable QoL. He already had a living will and health care power of attorney. He was currently "full code," meaning that he did not have a do-not-resuscitate (DNR) order, but after discussion the family agreed that attempting resuscitation on his death would be extremely unlikely to result in a tolerable QoL for him. The physician wrote a DNR order. During exploration of the question of whether or not to proceed with a prostate biopsy, his family stated that, even if the biopsy were positive for cancer, they would not want to put John through cancer treatment. They decided to cancel the biopsy.

(Continued)

CASE EXAMPLE 3.1. JOHN: ALZHEIMER'S DISEASE AND PALLIATIVE CARE *(Cont.)*

The occupational therapist's interventions were very helpful for the patient and his wife and resulted in increased medication compliance and safer bathing practices. Both the occupational therapist and the physician continued to see John regularly. Approximately 1 year after the initial occupational therapy assessment, his care team noted that his cognition had worsened. He now needed more supervision for even basic tasks such as brushing his teeth or taking out the trash. On one visit from family, he did not recognize his daughter.

Eighteen months after his initial visit, he was having trouble with the mechanics of toileting. He was continent of both bowel and bladder but sometimes could not find the toilet and one time defecated on the floor in the basement as a result of confusion. He had one episode in which he got out of the house and was wandering outside, but he was quickly found without injury. He also had one episode of delusional thinking. The family was working on getting him into adult day care to help ease the caregiving burden for his wife, who continued to get weaker.

At the 4-week follow up, John had incontinence of urine and frequently stool. He was talking less and having more delusions and hallucinations. The occupational therapist helped to educate Betty on and advocate for viable respite options and work on strategies to address his delusions and hallucinations. Noting John's rapid decline, the physician and occupational therapist revisited goals of care with the family and let them know that John was approaching eligibility for hospice. They discussed that service in detail and then let the family think and discuss it. They scheduled follow-up for 2 weeks later. By now, John was in adult day care 8 hours per day, and his wife's diagnosis had transformed from chronic leukemia to acute leukemia. His family had discussed hospice, and they wanted to proceed. He was admitted to hospice at home 2 days later. Twelve days after that he was transferred from home to a locked memory-care assisted living facility. His wife was admitted to hospice at home 2 months later and died 4 days after admission. By that time, John's memory loss had progressed to the point at which it was unclear whether he understood that she had died. He died peacefully in his assisted living facility about 11 months after hospice admission.

CASE EXAMPLE 3.2. DARLENE: ALZHEIMER'S DISEASE AND PALLIATIVE CARE

Darlene is a 73-year-old woman with advanced Alzheimer's disease. She had been working with an occupational therapist under the Skills2Care program for a few years. Her primary caregiver was her husband. They lived together in an independent living apartment on the grounds of a nursing home complex. Her husband's care for her was complicated by the fact that he had limb-girdle muscular dystrophy, so he often lacked the strength to safely transfer her or help her up after a fall. They primarily worked on strategies to make transfers safer and easier. The occupational therapist noted a recent decline in cognition and function and asked the palliative care physician to see her. On the physician's first visit, he found that Darlene was incontinent of bowel and bladder, and her speech was limited to fewer than five intelligible words in the course of a conversation. Her family noted that she would sometimes cry for no obvious reason. Her neurologist recently started her on quetiapine, a second-generation antipsychotic medication, to help with sleep and the crying spells. The palliative care physician noted that she had an extensive medication list, including multiple medications that were likely no longer providing any benefit. He discussed goals of care with her husband and daughters. They were clear that they wanted her to never feel alone and would like more time with her as long as it could be quality time. They felt that her current QoL was acceptable. She had a living will and a health care power of attorney. The family believed that she had a DNR order but, on closer examination, the physician found that they had misinterpreted a clause in her living will, a very common error. Her living will specified that she be made DNR if she was unresponsive and on life support, but she did not currently fit that condition, so she was actually full code. After discussion, the physician signed a DNR order. The family agreed to deprescribing any unneeded medications, so he stopped her cholesterol-lowering medication and four supplements.

The occupational therapist and physician continued to see Darlene regularly. Four months after the physician's initial contact with her, he was contacted by the occupational therapist, who had noticed a significant cognitive decline, even since their last visit, and was now questioning whether she was eligible for hospice. By this time, her neurologist had changed her antipsychotic first to risperidone, another second-generation antipsychotic, and then to thioridazine, an older, more sedating, first-generation antipsychotic. Both the occupational therapist and the physician noted that she was less interactive, sleepier, and eating and drinking less,

(Continued)

CASE EXAMPLE 3.2. DARLENE: ALZHEIMER'S DISEASE AND PALLIATIVE CARE *(Cont.)*

and her gait was much less steady. Both the occupational therapist and physician recommended transitioning to hospice, and her family agreed. On admission, the physician stopped her dementia medications, aspirin, and two more supplements. A month after hospice admission, Darlene was having more weakness and trouble standing. She was sometimes scooting on her bottom across the floor instead of standing. Her urine was strong-smelling, and she held her hands back as if she was experiencing pain in her flanks. With her history of frequent urinary tract infections, the physician started an antibiotic.

Two months later, Darlene's cognitive and functional abilities had worsened to the point that she was no longer able to communicate at all and could not walk independently. Her family noted that her QoL was so poor now that they wished her decline would accelerate so she would not suffer any longer. The physician discussed with them the option of not treating her next urinary tract infection. Antibiotics certainly have a place in comfort care, but they are not always aligned with a patient's goals. When a patient is trapped with an intolerable QoL, the question "Would treating this patient's infection and possibly prolonging their life be the best option for them?" needs to be asked. It can be a compassionate choice to allow an infection to progress untreated and simply maintain comfort. Darlene's team began working on moving her into long-term care. Five days after the move, she died peacefully in her room at the nursing home.

CASE EXAMPLE 3.3. DALE: STROKE AND PALLIATIVE CARE

Dale, age 74 years, suffered a massive hemorrhagic stroke at his rural home and was airlifted 300 miles to a large hospital with a neuro-critical care unit. He presented with right-side hemiparesis, aphasia, and dysphagia, in addition to intensive medical issues, including pneumonia.

Annie, an occupational therapist on the palliative care team, entered Dale's room in the neuro-critical care unit and found his wife and two adult children. She understood that this was a family in crisis—Dale's wife had driven 5 hours to the hospital, and his children had flown in. All were far from home and grappling with the unexpected shock of Dale's stroke and uncertainty about the future.

(Continued)

CASE EXAMPLE 3.3. DALE: STROKE *(Cont.)*

Annie warmly introduced herself and described her role as one of advocacy and support, explaining that palliative care was another layer of support that the hospital provided. She began the initial meeting by saying, "I want to understand who Dale is—the whole person, as you know him." Because Dale's alertness was minimal and he was unable to speak, Annie directed her questions to his family, asking about his roles, valued occupations, and personality. The family enjoyed talking about Dale as a real person, not just as a stroke patient hooked up to countless machines. Annie learned that Dale was a semiretired builder who loved working with his hands; an avid golfer, hunter, and runner; a beloved cross-country coach; and a husband, father, and grandfather. Through guided questions, she came to understand that Dale had a stubborn and determined personality, and he was socially engaged and active in many beloved occupational pursuits.

Annie brought up DNR orders, and the family agreed, because of Dale's strong-willed personality, to continue life-saving measures in the hope that rehabilitation could bring him a QoL he could tolerate. Although hopeful, the family was also realistic. Annie could see that they were distressed by their loved one's sudden incapacitation and immediate loss of valued roles and occupations. As goals for Dale were discussed, the family indicated that focused rehabilitation to attain QoL was most important.

Annie spent time with Dale and his family each day. She was wholly present, empathetic, and unrushed. When family members had medical questions, Annie ensured they received answers or visits from the physicians or therapists. Because she knew the family was in an unfamiliar city and cut off from their usual routines, she encouraged basic self-care, such as eating, sleeping, and breaks from Dale's bedside, and offered strategies to develop a healthy, balanced routine as they bounced from various hotels to the hospital and back.

As discharge came closer, the family felt the case manager was indifferent to Dale's placement in a rehabilitation facility. Rehabilitation and QoL were goals for Dale, but multiple facilities rejected his case because of the severity of the stroke. Annie assisted the case manager in pursuing other rehabilitation options, but more important, she gave a listening ear and practical support to Dale's overwhelmed, stressed wife. She described Annie as "the calm spot in the storm" and greatly valued the feeling that someone at the hospital was truly on her husband's side—as a person, not a case.

(Continued)

CASE EXAMPLE 3.3. DALE: STROKE *(Cont.)*

Ultimately, only one rehabilitation facility agreed to take Dale, and the partnership with the hospital, and Annie, ended. After 4 months of valiant effort in rehabilitation, and a couple of weeks of inpatient rehabilitation, Dale's improvement plateaued, and he disengaged. Wracked by nerve pain, spasticity, muscle contractions, dysphagia, depression, and hardly any ability to express himself, Dale's QoL was intolerable. He decided to stop rehabilitation efforts. The family supported his decision, and this autonomy—after months of being told what to do by therapists, nursing staff, and family members—did improve his QoL.

Although Dale qualified for hospice under Medicare because of his stroke, the closest hospice-certified, long-term-care facility was 80 miles away from home. He wanted to be in his own small town, so he was moved to a long-term-care facility there that did not have hospice services. His primary care physician took over palliative management of Dale's care by providing pain medications, assurance of his autonomy, and emotional support for his wife. When he was ready, after about 6 weeks receiving palliative care, Dale decided to stop the feeding tube. Several days later, Dale died.

Contributed by Ashley Hofmann. Used with permission.

Christian H. Jacobus, MD, FACEP, FAAHPM, is the Hospice Medical Director for Bridge Home Health and Hospice in Findlay, Ohio. He is board certified in both emergency medicine and hospice and palliative medicine. He loves his clinical practice but is also passionate about teaching, especially on the intersection of palliative care and the emergency department.

Lindsey Buddelmeyer, OTD, MOT, OTR/L, is the Leadership Education & Training Specialist at Blanchard Valley Health System in Findlay, Ohio. She has a personal and professional passion for advocating and working with the chronic disease community. Lindsey has been published and presented at both the state and national level during the past 10 years of her career. These experiences and platforms have included a wide range of community and professional organizations involving direct and indirect relations to palliative and hospice care.

REFERENCES

American Occupational Therapy Association. (2020). Occupational therapy practice framework: Domain and process (4th ed.). *American Journal of Occupational Therapy, 74*(Suppl. 2), 7412410010. https://doi.org/10.5014/ajot.2020.74S2001

Anderson, F., Downing, G. M., Hill, J., Casorso, L., & Lerch, N. (1996). Palliative Performance Scale (PPS): A new tool. *Journal of Palliative Care, 12*(1), 5–11. https://doi.org/10.1177/082585979601200102

Bakitas, M. A., Tosteson, T. D., Li, Z., Lyons, K. D., Hull, J. G., Li, Z., . . . Ahles, T. A. (2015). Early versus delayed initiation of concurrent palliative oncology care: Patient outcomes in the ENABLE III randomized controlled trial. *Journal of Clinical Oncology, 33,* 1438–1445. https://doi.org/10.1200/jco.2014.58.6362

Baum, A., Kaboli, P. J., & Schwartz, M. D. (2021). Reduced in-person and increased telehealth outpatient visits during the COVID-19 pandemic. *Annals of Internal Medicine, 174*(1), 129–131. https://doi.org/10.7326/m20-3026

Braus, N., Campbell, T. C., Kwekkeboom, K. L., Ferguson, S., Harvey, C., Krupp, A. E., . . . Ehlenbach, W. J. (2015). Prospective study of a proactive palliative care rounding intervention in a medical ICU. *Intensive Care Medicine, 42,* 54–62. https://doi.org/10.1007/s00134-015-4098-1

Bruera, E., Kuehn, N., Miller, M. J., Selmser, P., & Macmillan, K. (1991). The Edmonton Symptom Assessment System (ESAS): A simple method for the assessment of Palliative Care Patients. *Journal of Palliative Care, 7*(2), 6–9. https://doi.org/10.1177/082585979100700202

Casarett, D., Shreve, S., Luhrs, C., Lorenz, K., Smith, D., De Sousa, M., & Richardson, D. (2010). Measuring families' perceptions of care across a health care system: Preliminary experience with the Family Assessment of Treatment at End of Life Short Form (FATE-S). *Journal of Pain and Symptom Management, 40,* 801–809. https://doi.org/10.1016/j.jpainsymman.2010.03.019

Center to Advance Palliative Care. (2022). *About palliative care.* https://www.capc.org/about/palliative-care/

Clark, D. (1999). "Total pain," disciplinary power, and the body in the work of Cicely Saunders, 1958–1967. *Social Science & Medicine, 49*(6), 727–736. https://doi.org/10.1016/s0277-9536(99)00098-2

Coleman, E. A., Eilertsen, T. B., Kramer, A. M., Magid, D. J., Beck, A., & Conner, D. (2001). Reducing emergency visits in older adults with chronic illness: A randomized, controlled trial of group visits. *Effective Clinical Practice, 4*(2), 49–57.

Dionne-Odom, J. N., Azuero, A., Lyons, K. D., Hull, J. G., Tosteson, T., Li, Z., . . . Bakitas, M. A. (2015). Benefits of early versus delayed palliative care to informal family caregivers of patients with advanced cancer: Outcomes from the

ENABLE III randomized controlled trial. *Journal of Clinical Oncology, 33,* 1446–1452. https://doi.org/10.1200/jco.2014.58.7824

Ferrell, B., Sun, V., Hurria, A., Cristea, M., Raz, D. J., Kim, J. Y., . . . Koczywas, M. (2015). Interdisciplinary palliative care for patients with lung cancer. *Journal of Pain and Symptom Management, 50*(6), 758–767. https://doi.org/10.1016/j.jpainsymman.2015.07.005

Franklin, A., & Lovell, M. R. (2018). *Pain and pain management.* Springer.

Gade, G., Venohr, I., Conner, D., McGrady, K., Beane, J., Richardson, R. H., . . . Penna, R. D. (2008). Impact of an inpatient palliative care team: A randomized controlled trial. *Journal of Palliative Medicine, 11,* 180–190. https://doi.org/10.1089/jpm.2007.0055

Institute of Medicine. (1972). *Educating for the health team: Report of the Conference on the Interrelationships of Educational Programs for Health Professionals October 2–3, 1972.* National Academy of Sciences.

Jang, R. W., Krzyzanowska, M. K., Zimmermann, C., Taback, N., & Alibhai, S. M. (2015). Palliative care and the aggressiveness of end-of-life care in patients with advanced pancreatic cancer. *JNCI: Journal of the National Cancer Institute, 107*(3), dju424. https://doi.org/10.1093/jnci/dju424

Karnofsky, D. A., Abelmann, W. H., Craver, L. F., & Burchenal, J. H. (1948). The use of the nitrogen mustards in the palliative treatment of carcinoma. With particular reference to bronchogenic carcinoma. *Cancer, 1*(4), 634–656. https://doi.org/10.1002/1097-0142(194811)1:4<634::aid-cncr2820010410>3.0.co;2-l

Lustbader, D., Mudra, M., Romano, C., Lukoski, E., Chang, A., Mittelberger, J., . . . Cooper, D. (2017). The impact of a home-based palliative care program in an accountable care organization. *Journal of Palliative Medicine, 20*(1), 23–28. https://doi.org/10.1089/jpm.2016.0265

Maciejewski, M. L., Hammill, B. G., Bayliss, E. A., Ding, L., Voils, C. I., Curtis, L. H., Wang, V. (2017). Prescriber continuity and disease control of older adults. *Medical Care, 55*(4), 405–410. https://doi.org/10.1097/MLR.0000000000000658

May, P., Garrido, M. M., Cassel, J. B., Kelley, A. S., Meier, D. E., Normand, C., . . . Morrison, R. S. (2015). Prospective cohort study of hospital palliative care teams for inpatients with advanced cancer: Earlier consultation is associated with larger cost-saving effect. *Journal of Clinical Oncology, 33,* 2745–2752. https://doi.org/10.1200/jco.2014.60.2334

Morley, L., & Cashell, A. (2017). Collaboration in health care. *Journal of Medical Imaging Radiation Sciences, 48,* 207–216. http://dx.doi.org/10.1016/j.jmir.2017.02.071

Nasreddine, Z. S., Phillips, N. A., Bédirian, V., Charbonneau, S., Whitehead, V., Collin, I., Cummings, J. L., & Chertkow, H. (2005). The Montreal Cognitive Assessment, MoCA: A brief screening tool for mild cognitive impairment. *Journal of the American Geriatrics Society, 53*(4), 695–699. https://doi.org/10.1111/j.1532-5415.2005.53221.x

National Center for Chronic Disease Prevention. (2021). *About chronic diseases.* https://www.cdc.gov/chronicdisease/about/index.htm

Scheffey, C., Kestenbaum, M. G., Wachterman, M. W., Connor, S. R., Fine, P. G., Davis, M. S., & Muir, J. C. (2014). Clinic-based outpatient palliative care before hospice is associated with longer hospice length of service. *Journal of Pain and Symptom Management, 48,* 532–539. https://doi.org/10.1016/j.jpainsymman.2013.10.017

Stevens, D. W., & Bowman, B. (2020). *8 ways to keep your palliative care program off the chopping block.* Center to Advance Palliative Care. https://www.capc.org/blog/palliative-pulse-the-palliative-pulse-april-2018-palliative-care-program-off-chopping-block/

Sullivan, D. R., Chan, B., Lapidus, J. A., Ganzini, L., Hansen, L., Carney, P. A., . . . Slatore, C. G. (2019). Association of early palliative care use with survival and place of death among patients with advanced lung cancer receiving care in the Veterans Health Administration. *JAMA Oncology, 5,* 1702–1709. https://doi.org/10.1001/jamaoncol.2019.3105

Temel, J. S., Greer, J. A., Muzikansky, A., Gallagher, E. R., Admane, S., Jackson, V. A., . . . Lynch, T. J. (2010). Early palliative care for patients with metastatic non–small-cell lung cancer. *New England Journal of Medicine, 363,* 733–742. https://doi.org/10.1056/nejmoa1000678

Verberkt, C. A., van den Beuken-van Everdingen, M. H., Schols, J. M., Hameleers, N., Wouters, E. F., & Janssen, D. J. (2020). Effect of sustained-release morphine for refractory breathlessness in chronic obstructive pulmonary disease on health status: A randomized clinical trial. *JAMA Internal Medicine, 180,* 1306–1314. https://doi.org/10.1001/jamainternmed.2020.3134

4

Hospice and Occupational Therapy

HEATHER McKAY, PhD, OTR/L; CHRISTIAN H. JACOBUS, MD, FACEP, FAAHPM; and DAVID BENTHALL, MS, OTR/L

Learning Objectives

After completing this chapter, readers will be able to

- define the mission and philosophy of hospice care;
- recognize the basic elements of the Medicare hospice benefit, including reimbursement, regulatory guidelines, and implications for occupational therapy;
- understand occupational therapy's role in hospice care and strategies to enhance patients' participation in meaningful occupations at the end of life; and
- summarize the evidence from the scientific literature regarding the benefits of occupation and outcomes of occupational therapy for people nearing the end of life and their families.

Key Terms and Concepts

bereavement care
chronic disease
end-of-life care
end-of-life occupations
good death
hospice
hospice philosophy
interdisciplinary team approach
life-limiting illness
Medicare hospice benefit
occupational participation
principal diagnosis
respite care
routine care

quality of life
terminal illness
value-based care

In Case Example 4.1, Sara is just one of a growing population who receive hospice care in the United States annually. The number of hospice patients rose from 1.3 million in 2015 to 1.6 million by 2019 (National Hospice and Palliative Care Organization [NHPCO], 2020). Of all Medicare decedents in 2019, 51.6% were enrolled in hospice at the time of their death. As the overall age of the population increases, the demand for hospice care is expected to continue the same upward trend. Today, hospice agencies are reaching more families in their time of need. However, the facts and figures on who receives hospice care and when in the United States suggest that the current growth rate may still be lagging behind a much larger need, particularly for people with a noncancer condition (Cagle et al., 2020). Serious concerns exist about equal access to comprehensive end-of-life care across diagnostic groups, geographic areas, and racial and ethnic populations.

Moreover, hospice professionals continue to express concerns about the number of people accessing their hospice benefit in the last stage of their illness. Experts believe that when the transition to hospice is delayed unnecessarily or skipped altogether, patients and families miss a critical opportunity for personally meaningful end-of-life care. In 2018, more than a quarter (27.9%) of beneficiaries received care for 7 days or less, which is not considered enough time for patients to receive the full benefit of person- and family-centered services available through hospice (NHPCO, 2020). The advantages of longer hospice enrollment (≥30 days) have been well documented, including reduced costs, greater patient goal attainment, effective pain management, higher family-reported satisfaction, and a greater likelihood that the patient can die in their preferred place (Kumar et al., 2017; Mulville et al., 2019). Further inquiry is needed to examine the underuse of hospice services in the United States to better guide policy, research, and practice. Although all eligible patients may not elect hospice enrollment, high-quality hospice care must be accessible to all eligible patients and families in a timely manner.

As the needs of people with terminal illness grow, so too will the demand for high-quality end-of-life care that is more effective, efficient,

CASE EXAMPLE 4.1. SARA: PART 1

Sara was an 80-year-old retired schoolteacher who had been coping with advanced congestive heart failure (CHF) for more than 5 years. After a fall at home, Sara was hospitalized with worsening CHF symptoms and a broken clavicle. Upon discharge from the hospital, she transitioned to a skilled nursing facility for subacute rehabilitation. Sara and the interdisciplinary team initially expected that she would regain strength and functional skills before returning home, where she lived with her daughter and grandson. However, Sara's progress in rehabilitation stalled, and she required significant assistance with most ADLs and IADLs.

Sara was working with the occupational therapist on ADL retraining one morning when her thoughts shifted to her emerging concerns, priorities, and goals of care. Sara was looking in the bathroom mirror when she said tearfully, "Things seem to be getting worse, not better." The therapist paused the grooming activity and reflected with Sara on the symptoms that were hampering her ADL performance, including fatigue, shortness of breath, pain, trouble swallowing, and difficulty thinking. The therapist noticed that Sara's spirits lifted when they spoke about her most valued occupation, spending time with her grandson. The therapist used empathy, active listening, clinical reasoning, and collaborative problem solving as the two clarified Sara's main concern and possible solutions together.

Sara: "I fear that I'm wasting valuable time trying to do things that are no longer possible for me."

OT: "It sounds like you're thinking of other, more important things you would rather be doing these days."

Sara: "Yes. I want to maximize my time with my family. I can't do that while they're at home, and I'm here. I've noticed during their visits that I'm too tired to do things with them after struggling to do everything for myself each day. . . . I feel my body failing, and I want to spend my limited time and energy on making positive memories with my daughter and grandson. If receiving more help with these self-care activities left me with the energy to read him a bedtime story, to me, that's time and energy well spent."

OT: "Oh, Sara, I can tell you've been doing some real soul-searching, and you have a positive outlook on the rest of your life. It sounds like you want to make the most of your remaining time, which aligns with the hospice philosophy that the last chapter of life is just as important as the earlier chapters. Have you ever spoken with your doctor about hospice?"

Sara: "I do want to make the most of every day I have left, and I believe I can only do that at home. I've known friends and family who received hospice in their homes, but

(Continued)

CASE EXAMPLE 4.1. SARA: PART 1 *(Cont.)*

I thought you had to be on your deathbed to receive that help. I know that I want hospice, for my family's sake and mine, but I don't know when hospice could help."

OT: "It sounds like your goals of care are evolving, and it's a perfect time to talk with the whole team about the road ahead, including hospice. I believe if we put more heads together, we could create a plan that includes the right care for you and your family at the right time. Would you be willing to meet with the team to talk more about goals of care and possible options?"

Sara: "That's exactly what I want and need to do as soon as possible. I appreciate your willingness to listen and think through this problem with me."

Occupational therapy practitioners often encounter opportunities for critical conversations because of the intimate nature of their work. Such opportunities may be in the context of a personal care activity or a moment of fun during a leisure activity when patients feel most ready to speak about deeply meaningful occupational roles or their vision of themselves and their future. In this case, the occupational therapist working in the rehabilitation setting noticed a window for a timely conversation that set Sara's care plan on a new trajectory. Thanks to the therapist's advocacy, Sara and her daughter were able to meet together with the interdisciplinary team. They learned that Sara was eligible for her hospice benefit, and the doctor explained more about the signs of end-stage heart failure that were the basis of that determination. The family decided that traditional rehabilitation goals were no longer their priority and going home with support from hospice was their preferred option.

The case leads to some critical thinking questions:

1. Was the occupational therapist reasoning and responding appropriately by broaching the subject of hospice and advocating for a care plan meeting according to Sara's dying wishes?
2. What evidence exists to support the benefits of occupation for patients nearing the end of life and their families?
3. As Sara's functional skills continue to decline, does Sara qualify for continued occupational therapy services under hospice? If so, who initiates that occupational therapy referral, and how does the therapist's focus shift in the hospice model?

and satisfying to patients and their families. This leads to the following questions:

- What is occupational therapy's role in end-of-life care?
- What shifts are necessary in occupational therapy's focus when the patient's independence and functional performance skills are expected to decline?

- What do patients stand to gain from occupational therapy as they near the end of life?

This chapter provides a background on hospice, aligns occupational therapy's distinct value with the hospice philosophy, presents the current evidence for occupational therapy in end-of-life care, and explores some potential reasons why occupational therapy remains underused in this emerging practice area and possible solutions to close the service gap. This chapter answers many important questions about occupational therapy and hospice—who, what, when, where, and why—and lays important groundwork for Chapter 6, "Delivering Occupational Therapy Services in Hospice Care," in which we explain step-by-step how occupational therapy practitioners work in this emerging practice area.

Hospice Background

DEFINITIONS

End-of-life care is the general term used to describe the support and medical care delivered during the months, weeks, days, and even moments leading up to a person's death (National Institute on Aging, 2021). ***Hospice*** is considered the blue-ribbon model for quality, compassionate end-of-life care for people facing a terminal illness. Encompassed in the hospice model is expert medical care, pain management, and emotional and spiritual support expressly tailored to the dying person's needs and wishes. Hospice also provides supportive services to the patient's family before, during, and after their loved one's death. Hospice is a holistic patient- and family-centered approach to health care in the patient's final chapter of life (Centers for Medicare & Medicaid Services [CMS], 2021a).

HISTORICAL PERSPECTIVE

The word *hospice* comes from the Latin *hospitum,* meaning "guest house, hospitality" (NHPCO, 2022). The oldest concept of hospice appeared throughout Europe in the 11th century as a resting place for ill or weary travelers, usually operated by monastic orders. In these resting places, monks or nuns provided housing for travelers, nursing care for the sick, and spiritual support to help people continue on their journey. Over the centuries, the concept of hospice evolved to mean care for people who were sick and alone in the community. In 1842, Madame Jeanne Garnier used the term *hospice* more explicitly to mean care for the dying (NHPCO, 2022).

Hospice in the modern sense of the word, as a philosophy of care for dying patients and their families, came to the United States in the late 20th century, promoted by the English physician (and former nurse and social worker) Dame Cicely Saunders (NHPCO, 2022). In 1963, Dame Saunders presented a speech on specialized care for the dying during a conference at Yale University, hosted by Florence Wald, dean of the Yale School of Nursing. Dame Saunders asserted about people nearing the end of life, "You matter because of who you are. You matter to the last moment of your life, and we will do all we can, not only to help you die peacefully but also to live until you die" (American Cancer Society, 2019, para. 1).

Dame Saunders championed comfort care for dying patients, including medical, social, psychological, and spiritual support, and ultimately founded the first modern hospice, St. Christopher's, in London in 1967 (NHPCO, 2022). After visiting the London hospice, Saunders's colleague, Florence Wald, along with two pediatricians and a chaplain, founded Connecticut Hospice in Bradford, Connecticut, in 1974, and they hosted the first National Symposium on Hospice Care in Connecticut the following year. In 1978, the National Hospice Organization (NHO) was established to promote the concept of hospice care. Throughout the late 1970s to 1980s, NHO collaborated with federal agencies and determined that hospice was a viable model that could potentially provide more humane and cost-effective care for Americans dying of terminal illness. For more than a decade, government agencies studied pilot hospice programs to clarify the scope and cost of the model; developed standards for accreditation for hospice agencies; and instilled the hospice benefit in Medicare, Medicaid, and private insurance plans. This movement in support of death with dignity happened against the backdrop of the AIDS pandemic of the 1980s (NHPCO, 2022).

HOSPICE PHILOSOPHY

At the heart of hospice is a belief that compassionate care for people in the last stage of an incurable disease can enhance their ***quality of life*** (QoL) and help people live more fully and comfortably in their remaining time. Hospice acknowledges that QoL is a subjective, multidimensional evaluation of how good or satisfactory one's life is. In the context of hospice, patient-valued aspects of QoL include physical, cognitive, emotional, social, and spiritual well-being; personal autonomy; health care provision; and preparation for death (McCaffrey et al., 2016). Hospice acknowledges that human growth and development can be a lifelong process and seeks to preserve and promote an individual's and family's inherent potential for growth in the last chapter of life (NHPCO, 2018). Thus, the hospice philosophy accepts death as the natural final phase of life; it affirms life and neither hastens nor postpones death.

Hospice philosophy encompasses holistic symptom control and meeting the emotional, social, spiritual, and functional needs of the patient and family. For example, when a patient reports they are in pain, the source of that pain could be feelings of social isolation, unresolved interpersonal issues, or existential distress, to name a few. To focus only on the physical dimensions of suffering is to ignore other potential root causes responsible for a significant amount of distress. Therefore, according to the hospice philosophy, optimal comfort care means addressing all causes of suffering (this is known as a palliative approach to care and is addressed in more detail in Chapter 3, "Palliative Care and Occupational Therapy"). As such, electing hospice does not mean giving up or doing less; when a person elects a hospice benefit, they often receive different services, not fewer, with an emphasis on social, psychological, and spiritual aspects of care (American Cancer Society, 2019). This approach to care is inherently patient and family centered because hospice identifies the patient and family or caregiver as the collective unit of care. For a hospice patient, the family may include blood relatives, friends, or anyone identified by the patient as their inner circle.

Finally, the hospice philosophy asserts that these goals can only be accomplished through an ***interdisciplinary team approach*** (NHPCO, 2018). In hospice, the interdisciplinary collaboration involves a diverse group of physicians, nurses, home health aides, social workers, counselors, chaplains, therapists, and trained volunteers working together to address each hospice patient's and family's needs.

Distinguishing Palliative Care and Hospice

For many patients and their families, hearing the words *palliative care* or *hospice* may be upsetting, confusing, and even stigmatizing. The confusion grows when health care workers or laypeople mistakenly use the terms interchangeably. As stated in Chapter 3, although palliative care and hospice are similar, the two care models have important differences. Helping people understand the meaning of and differences between palliative care and hospice can help patients and families choose for themselves the right care at the right time.

Hospice is a subsection of palliative care for people of any age with a life-limiting illness for whom further curative measures are no longer desired or appropriate (Hospice Foundation of America [HFA], 2018b). Hospice and palliative care both aim to provide a better QoL and relief from symptoms and side effects for people with serious illnesses. Both have special care teams that address a person's physical, emotional, mental, social, and spiritual needs. It is accurate to say that hospice takes a palliative, not curative, approach to care in the final stage of a disease. All hospice care is palliative care because it focuses on symptom management, but not all palliative care includes hospice (HFA, 2018b). Hospice differs from other palliative care services in four ways: (1) timing, (2) approach to curative treatments, (3) the hospice team's role, and (4) bereavement care.

TIMING

The first distinguishing factor between hospice and other palliative care is timing. Hospice is reserved for the terminal stage of a patient's condition (NHPCO, 2021). A patient is eligible for hospice when their life expectancy is 6 months or less, given the normal course of the diagnosis. The patient is then said to be living with a ***terminal*** or ***life-limiting illness.*** Palliative care, however, can be initiated at any time during a serious illness or ***chronic disease*** (a disease that persists for a year or longer that requires ongoing medical attention, limits daily life activities, or both; Centers for Disease Control and Prevention, 2022).

APPROACH TO CURATIVE TREATMENTS

Second, the two services differ in how they approach curative treatments. Typically, hospice is provided when no curative treatment is being given—because a curative treatment does not exist, the patient opted out of it, or curative treatment for comorbidities is deemed inappropriate because it would only prolong suffering. In contrast, palliative care can coexist with curative treatments at any point in the disease course. There are two exceptions to this rule, though. The first is that since 2009, the U.S. Department of Veterans Affairs (VA) has allowed patients with incurable diseases to receive disease-directed therapy (e.g., immunotherapy, chemotherapy, radiation, intravenous furosemide) while also paying for hospice, what the VA calls "concurrent care hospice." The VA instituted concurrent care in response to the realization that only 5% of veterans who died received hospice support. So, the VA removed the requirement that the veteran forgo curative therapy to receive hospice care, avoiding the "terrible choice" between disease treatment and home-based supportive care (Broderick, 2020). The second exception to the rule is that children (up to age 21 years) with federally funded insurance such as Medicare or Medicaid can receive hospice and life-prolonging care at the same time under a section of the Patient Protection and Affordable Care Act (P. L. 111-148) titled "Concurrent Care for Children" (Lindley et al., 2020). For both exceptions, the patient must have a life expectancy of 6 months or less. These exceptions mean that, in certain cases, a patient can be on hospice and receive regular rehabilitative services, chemotherapy, radiation, dialysis, and other potentially life-prolonging care.

Exceptions to the curative treatment rule are likely to be more common in the coming years because national data suggest that concurrent care could cost less, despite affording the patient access to disease-targeted treatments simultaneously with their full hospice benefit (Mor et al., 2019). Researchers have attributed the lower cost of some concurrent care to the lower likelihood that patients receiving support from the hospice team would need aggressive treatment or emergency care in the intensive care unit (Mor et al., 2019). In 2022, the CMS (2022b) evaluated a pilot program called the Medicare Care Choices Model (MCCM) that offered beneficiaries the option of receiving hospice services at the end of life without forgoing payment for treatment of their terminal condition. Researchers wanted to know whether concurrent care improved the quality of care, increased beneficiaries' satisfaction, and reduced Medicare expenditures (CMS, 2022b). More than 6,000 beneficiaries (of 6,427 participants, 72% had terminal cancer) enrolled in the model at 141 participating hospices over a 5.5-year period from January 2016 to June 2021 (the model ended December 31, 2021). The outcomes supported the model. Specifically, MCCM beneficiaries were more likely to elect their hospice benefit when not forced to forgo disease-targeted treatment, less likely to use hospital services and other health care services, and more likely to receive better-quality end-of-life care in the period between enrollment in MCCM and death. Researchers believed that earlier hospice enrollment drove the decreased need for resource-intensive services and lower Medicare expenditures (CMS, 2022b).

HOSPICE TEAM'S ROLE

The hospice team's role is a third factor distinguishing it from palliative care. The hospice team coordinates and supervises all of the patient's care 24 hours a day, 7 days a week, and hospice care includes some special services not included in palliative care. For example, many families are relieved to learn that in addition to the hospice team's scheduled visits, a hospice nurse is available around the clock to address emerging questions and concerns. Under the hospice benefit, the on-call nurse can make additional unscheduled visits as needed for problem solving, night or day. Respite care is another service unique to the hospice benefit. ***Respite care*** is short-term relief for in-home hospice caregivers. When the hospice team determines that a family caregiver needs a break or the patient needs short-term inpatient services, the patient's hospice benefit will pay for the transport and short stay in a facility.

BEREAVEMENT CARE

Finally, hospice is the only medical service model that includes ***bereavement care*** (HFA, 2018a). Hospice addresses grief and bereavement needs starting at the time of admission and continues for 13 months after the patient's death or longer, if needed. Anticipatory grief services are provided to help the patient, family, caregivers, and other people identified by the patient cope with the losses that occur throughout the dying process. Bereavement services are provided before and after the death, based on a comprehensive bereavement assessment, including risk factors for complicated grief, social support, concurrent life stressors, relationship with the deceased, and other relevant factors (NHPCO, 2018).

Hospice Eligibility

Occupational therapy practitioners field common questions about end-of-life care, including who qualifies for hospice and how they connect with the service. Patients qualify for hospice when two providers (the referring provider and the hospice medical director) determine that their life expectancy is 6 months or less, given the usual course of their disease (i.e., the person is living with a terminal or life-limiting illness), and the patient or family have decided that curative treatments are no longer either desired or appropriate (see Case Example 4.2).

Life is unpredictable, and no one can know for certain exactly what will happen in a person's disease trajectory. However, this very uncertainty is why creating opportunities for early discussion regarding end-of-life care is so important. Determining whether or when someone is eligible for hospice and their care preferences requires communication among the patient, family, and entire health care team, but too frequently these conversations do not occur. Often, patients and relatives will wait for end-of-life care topics to be raised by clinicians, whereas clinicians will wait for the patient or family to open the conversation—a common scenario captured by Almack et al. (2012) in their article titled "After You." Because timely and appropriate identification of hospice-eligible patients increases the likelihood that they and their families will benefit from compassionate, comprehensive end-of-life care, the CMS has published general guidelines to aid health care workers and the public

CASE EXAMPLE 4.2. SARA: PART 2

The occupational therapist had correctly reasoned and advocated for the care plan meeting to discuss hospice eligibility and potential care transition on the basis of Sara's clinical history and her wish to shift away from rehabilitation interventions that felt fruitless to her in pursuit of her new QoL goals. During the meeting, the nurse practitioner at the rehab facility determined that Sara's CHF was in the terminal stage. In conversation with the team and her family, Sara confirmed she was ready to let go of life-prolonging curative treatments because they were no longer effective or satisfying to her and impeded other goals that were more important to Sara and her family at this time.

The nurse practitioner sent the referral to Sara's hospice of choice, where the medical director agreed that her diagnosis of CHF was terminal and Sara was eligible for hospice (two providers signed for the hospice admission). Sara's hospice benefits began the same day. With support from hospice, Sara transitioned home with family as she had hoped.

in understanding when a person qualifies for hospice care (CMS, 2021b). Hospice should be considered if a person meets two or more of the following general criteria:

- progression of disease as documented by worsening clinical status, symptoms, signs, and laboratory results
- dependence in two or more ADLs (e.g., feeding, ambulation, continence, transfers, bathing, dressing)
- shortness of breath or fatigue at rest or after minimal exertion
- increasing emergency department visits or hospitalizations
- decrease in cognitive function
- critical nutrition impairment (i.e., 10% weight loss in 6 months)
- impaired functional status as indicated by Karnofsky Performance Status (KPS; Karnofsky & Burchenal, 1949) or Palliative Performance Scale (PPS: Anderson et al., 1996) score of <70% (some disease-specific guidelines establish a lower qualifying KPS or PPS score)
- progressive decline in Functional Assessment Staging Tool (Reisberg, 1984) for dementia (score of ≥7A)
- progressive Stage 3–4 pressure ulcer despite optimal care
- decreased activity tolerance
- multiple falls with injury
- other comorbid conditions.

Common Conditions

It is common for patients nearing the end of life to have more than one serious health condition. Therefore, the ***principal diagnosis***—the condition that qualifies the person for their hospice benefit—is the condition that contributes the most to the patient's limited life expectancy (NHPCO, 2021). Specific diagnoses are collapsed into major disease groupings, and CMS (2021b) provides diagnosis-specific criteria (see Table 4.1 on p. 86) to help health care providers and the general public know when these common conditions are considered terminal. Although only a physician can determine whether a patient meets the qualifications for hospice admission, any health care worker who recognizes signs of end-stage disease may be instrumental in starting the collaborative conversation about adding hospice care at the right time. In addition to the principal diagnosis, a person's functional decline can also indicate hospice eligibility. For example, marked decreases in weight, weakness, fatigue, cognition, mobility, and ability to complete ADLs can support a person's hospice eligibility if these functional changes are determined to be irreversible and consistent with the principal diagnosis.

More than other health care providers, occupational therapy practitioners may be more attuned to changing levels of function when working with patients in different practice settings and can utilize their clinical reasoning to support and advocate for timely end-of-life care conversations and hospice referrals on the basis of their clinical assessment of the patient. The consensus is that the best outcomes for patients and their families are achieved when conversations about end-of-life wishes are started sooner, rather than later, while the patient still has the capacity to participate in their own care decisions (Baxter et al., 2022; Brighton & Bristowe, 2016).

If the patient has lost capacity, the benefits of proactive end-of-life conversations extend to family members and surrogate decision makers prior to the death and throughout their bereavement period. Initiating such conversations before the patient is imminently dying can enable the family to make the most of the time left, use the full range of hospice services, and prepare for the person's death while also maintaining hope (Brighton & Bristowe, 2016). The information in Table 4.1 is intended to boost occupational therapy practitioners' general awareness of signs that their patients may be eligible for hospice and provide terminology to help practitioners talk about end-of-life care options with patients, families, and teammates proactively.

A common misconception is that hospice is only for cancer patients, but patients with a life expectancy of less than 6 months are eligible. In fact, cancer as a whole has been steadily declining as a principal diagnosis among Medicare patients in hospice, down from 22% in 2002 to 4.9% in 2019. In 2019, more Medicare hospice patients had a principal diagnosis of Alzheimer's disease, dementia, or Parkinson's disease than of any other disease (20.9%). Lung disease (7.1%), heart disease (6.4%), and stroke (5.4%) were the next most common conditions among Medicare beneficiaries receiving hospice in 2019 (NHPCO, 2021).

Deciding if or when to forgo or stop life-prolonging treatments or procedures in exchange for different QoL interventions is a difficult choice for many patients and their families. Some patients and families struggle

TABLE 4.1. Diagnosis-Specific Hospice Eligibility Guidelines

Disease	Guidelines
Heart disease	Consider hospice if the patient meets both Criteria 1 and 2. Factors from Criterion 3 will add eligibility support. 1. Patient is or has already been optimally treated for heart disease or is not a candidate for a surgical procedure or has declined a procedure. 2. Patient is classified as New York Heart Association Class IV and may have significant symptoms of heart failure or angina at rest. Significant congestive heart failure may be documented by an ejection fraction of ≤20%. 3. Patient has treatment-resistant symptomatic supraventricular or ventricular arrhythmias, prior cardiac arrest, prior unexplained syncope, or other complications.
Cancer	Consider hospice if the patient exhibits either Criterion 1 or 2: 1. Disease with distant metastases 2. Progression from an earlier stage of the disease to metastatic disease with either a. continued decline despite optimal treatment or b. patient no longer wishes to pursue aggressive chemotherapy or immunotherapy *Note.* Certain cancers with poor prognosis (e.g., small cell lung cancer, brain cancer, pancreatic cancer) may qualify for hospice earlier than outlined in the criteria in this section.

(Continued)

TABLE 4.1. Diagnosis-Specific Hospice Eligibility Guidelines *(Cont.)*

Disease	Guidelines
Alzheimer's disease and related disorders	Consider hospice if the patient exhibits all of the following criteria: 1. Stage 7 or beyond on the Functional Assessment Staging Scale 2. Unable to ambulate without assistance 3. Unable to dress without assistance 4. Unable to bathe without assistance 5. Urinary and fecal incontinence, intermittent or constant 6. No consistently meaningful verbal communication: stereotypical phrases only or the ability to speak is limited to six or fewer intelligible words 7. Additional life-threatening complications within the past 12 months (e.g., recurrent pneumonia, upper urinary tract infection, sepsis, antibiotic-resistant fever, Stage 3–4 decubitus ulcer, significant weight loss in the past 6 months) *Note.* This section is specific to Alzheimer's disease and related disorders and is not specific to other types of dementia, such as multi-infarct dementia.

(Continued)

TABLE 4.1. Diagnosis-Specific Hospice Eligibility Guidelines *(Cont.)*

Disease	Guidelines
Stroke and coma	Consider hospice if the patient meets both Criteria 1 and 2 after a stroke: 1. KPS or PPS score of 40% or less 2. Inability to maintain hydration and caloric intake, along with weight loss >10% in the past 6 months, serum albumin <2.5 g/dL, pulmonary aspiration, or dysphagia severe enough to prevent the patient from receiving food and fluids necessary to sustain life Consider hospice if the patient meets any 3 of the following criteria on Day 3 of the coma: 1. Abnormal brainstem response 2. Absent verbal response 3. Absent withdrawal response to pain 4. Serum creatinine >1.5 mg/dl. Consider hospice if the patient has had medical complications, in the context of progressive clinical decline, within the previous 12 months, that support a terminal prognosis: 1. Aspiration pneumonia 2. Upper urinary tract infection 3. Sepsis 4. Stage 3–4 decubitus ulcers 5. Fever recurrent after antibiotics

(Continued)

TABLE 4.1. Diagnosis-Specific Hospice Eligibility Guidelines *(Cont.)*

Disease	Guidelines
Pulmonary or lung disease	Consider hospice if the patient meets both Criteria 1 and 2. Factors from Criterion 3 will add eligibility support. 1. Severe chronic lung disease with disabling dyspnea at rest, poorly responsive to bronchodilators, and increasing pulmonary infections or respiratory failure 2. Hypoxemia at rest on room air, as evidenced by pO2 ≤55 mmHg, oxygen saturation ≤88%; or hypercapnia, as evidenced by pCO2 ≥50 mmHg 3. Right heart failure due to pulmonary disease, progressive weight loss over the past 6 months, or resting tachycardia >100/min.
Liver disease	Consider hospice if the patient meets both Criteria 1 and 2. Factors from Criterion 3 will add eligibility support. 1. Prothrombin time prolonged more than 5 seconds over control or international normalized ratio >1.5 and serum albumin <2.5 g/dL 2. End-stage liver disease with ascites, bacterial peritonitis, hepatorenal syndrome, hepatic encephalopathy, or variceal bleeding 3. Progressive malnutrition, muscle wasting, continued alcoholism, hepatocellular carcinoma, or hepatitis B or C

(Continued)

TABLE 4.1. Diagnosis-Specific Hospice Eligibility Guidelines *(Cont.)*

Disease	Guidelines
Renal or kidney disease	Consider hospice if the patient meets Criterion 1 and either Criterion 2 or 3. Factors from Criterion 4 will add eligibility support. 1. Not seeking dialysis or renal transplant or discontinuing dialysis 2. Creatinine clearance glomerular filtration rate <15 ml/min 3. Serum creatinine >8.0 mg/dL (>6.0 mg/dL for persons with diabetes) 4. Signs and symptoms of renal failure or comorbid conditions such as malignancy, cardiac disease, liver disease, gastrointestinal bleeding, and sepsis, among others
ALS	Consider hospice if the patient meets Criterion 1, 2, or 3: 1. Critically impaired breathing capacity, as indicated by vital capacity <30%, dyspnea at rest, and patient declines mechanical ventilation or uses it for comfort measures only 2. Rapid progression of ALS and critical nutritional impairment 3. Rapid progression of ALS and life-threatening complications (e.g., recurrent pneumonia, upper urinary tract infection, sepsis, antibiotic-resistant fever, Stage 3–4 decubitus ulcer)

(Continued)

TABLE 4.1. Diagnosis-Specific Hospice Eligibility Guidelines *(Cont.)*

Disease	Guidelines
HIV disease	Consider hospice if the patient meets both Criterion 1 and 2. Factors from Criterion 3 will add eligibility support. 1. CD4+ count 100,000 copies/ml, plus systemic lymphoma, treatment-resistant bacterial infection, renal failure, or other life-threatening complication 2. Decreased performance status, as measured by the KPS scale, of ≤50% 3. Other life-threatening comorbidities such as AIDS-related dementia, congestive heart failure, and liver disease, among others

Note. ALS = amyotrophic lateral sclerosis; KPS = Karnofsky Performance Status; pCO2 = partial pressure of carbon dioxide; pO2 = partial pressure of oxygen; PPS = Palliative Performance Scale.

with questions such as "Am I giving up hope?" "Should we be fighting harder?" and "How will I know when it's time to let go?" All of these questions are complicated by cultural norms and societal expectations (e.g., a patient with cancer may feel pressure to continue treatment when praised for their warriorlike strength; a family member may fear judgment if they refuse life-prolonging treatment for a loved one, even when their loved one's wishes for a comfortable, natural death are clear).

Another hospice myth is that electing hospice means that a person is giving up and losing hope. The truth is that the patient's or family's definition of hope can change over time as the disease progresses. A review of the literature found that patients can maintain hope while also acknowledging their terminal prognosis. Initially, they may hope for a cure, but as medical options are exhausted and symptoms progress, they may hope to live longer than expected, enjoy a good QoL, achieve personal goals, or have a peaceful death (Clayton et al., 2008). Many may feel hopeful about leaving a legacy for their family. Understanding the many facets of hope can help clinicians see it as essential in end-of-life care and nurture hope for their patients, families, and themselves (Szabat & Knox, 2021).

Keep in mind that hospice is about caring, not curing, and all of its services are focused on the dying person and the grieving family's unique experience. Ongoing conversations about goals of care, starting as soon as a serious illness is identified, can ensure that patients and their families promptly receive care that is concordant with their values, goals, priorities, and preferences (Baxter et al., 2022). Even at the end of life, families and hospice caregivers never give up caring for the dying person, even if medical resources to cure or alter the course of illness have been exhausted. Hospice is both medical and supportive care with the goal of comfort and dignity (HFA, 2018a).

Although eligible patients and families have the greatest chance to maximize their hospice benefits if services are started early, even a short period of hospice support can make a positive difference for the patient and family. Sometimes hospice admission happens at the very end of the person's life. Although longer stays are generally thought to be of greater benefit to patients and families, even last-minute support by a hospice professional can ease the person's death and afford the family extensive bereavement services after the death that could make a positive difference in how they carry on with life after a significant loss. When time is of the essence, it is important to remember that anyone, including occupational therapy practitioners, other health care providers, or family members, can start a conversation about hospice care and initiate a hospice referral for anyone with any life-threatening illness (HFA, 2018a). Figure 4.1 illustrates that in 2019, fewer than 25% of patients received hospice for 6 months or longer. Most patients had relatively short stays, reinforcing the concerns about potential late hospice enrollment and the need for earlier end-of-life care conversations. In 2019, approximately one-quarter of hospice decedents were enrolled during the last week of life, and half of them received hospice for 18 days or less (NHPCO, 2021).

Locations of Care

Hospice cares for people wherever they are at the end of life (NHPCO, 2021). The location of care will differ depending on the person's preferences, needs, or choices. Some people may want to be at home when they die, and others may prefer to seek treatment in a hospital or facility in their final days. As their needs change, hospice patients may change locations without interruption in their hospice services. Hospice workers, including occupational therapy practitioners, can be instrumental in

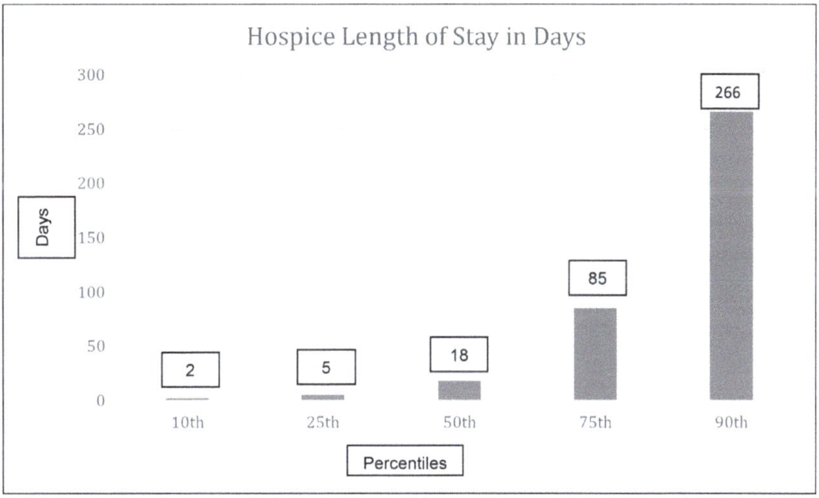

Figure 4.1 Days of hospice care patients received in 2019.

Source. Medicare Payment Advisory Commission (2021).

facilitating these transitions and helping people settle more comfortably in the new place. The majority of hospice patients receive services in the place they call home (NHPCO, 2021), which may be a private residence, nursing home, or another residential facility. Hospice is also provided in inpatient settings, including free-standing hospice facilities (sometimes referred to as hospice homes) and hospitals (NHPCO, 2021).

Regulatory Guidelines and Payment

MEDICARE HOSPICE BENEFIT

According to the NHPCO (2018), Medicare is the primary health insurer for more than 80% of people who die every year. The majority of hospice services are primarily reimbursed by Medicare and Medicaid through the ***Medicare hospice benefit*** unless otherwise covered via private health insurance. The Medicare hospice benefit was initially approved by the U.S. Congress in 1982. It sets the standard for hospice care in the United States and is the model for hospice benefits for other government and private insurance plans. Only care provided by a Medicare-certified hospice is covered under the Medicare hospice benefit (CMS, 2022a). A hospice agency must follow rules and regulations known as Medicare hospice conditions of participation to be Medicare certified and accept Medicare dollars (NHPCO, 2018).

In addition, NHPCO's Standards of Practice outline core components of quality by which an agency's entire operation is evaluated, including clinical and nonclinical operations (NHPCO, 2018). The Standards of Practice assist hospices in meeting the Medicare hospice conditions of participation that require Medicare-certified agencies to implement and maintain a quality assessment performance improvement (QAPI) process for their organization. The Standards of Practice provide a framework for developing and implementing QAPI, so they reflect hospice's commitment to continuously improve the care of patients and their families (NHPCO, 2018).

Hospices are paid on a per-diem basis, whether the payor is Medicare, Medicaid, or a private insurance company. A per-diem payment model means the agency receives a certain dollar amount from insurance for every day that a patient receives their service. Hospice agencies are required to provide nursing and aide services, social work, spiritual care, therapy services, bereavement support, medical equipment, most medications, and volunteer services as needed for each patient. The per-diem hospice rate varies depending on the intensity of care needed. The payment rate is higher in the first 60 days of service, decreases during the middle of the patient's care, and increases again in the final few days of care when the patient is actively dying. The per-diem reimbursement rate is also higher when a patient needs more intense inpatient care or inpatient-level care at home.

The per-diem payment model incentivizes hospice agencies to be quality minded and cost conscious (the per-diem model rewards the hospice agency for effectiveness and efficiency). The hospice per-diem model is different from a fee-for-service model in which an agency bills insurance for every service they provide (fee-for-service models reward providers or organizations for the volume of services provided). The per-diem payment system is considered to be more value based. In general, value-based care models (promoting quality over quantity of services) are emerging across health care to replace traditional fee-for-service models (LaPointe, 2022). ***Value-based care*** seeks to advance the Quadruple Aim consisting of enhanced patient experiences, improved clinical outcomes, reduced health care costs, and improved clinician experience (Foerster, 2020; LaPointe, 2022). As such, hospice is seen as an early leader in the value-based movement because it has been accountable for cost controls and quality gains longer than other areas of health care that operate under a traditional fee-for-service model. The goal of value-based care is ambitious but straightforward: Replace the nation's reliance on fragmented, fee-for-service care with comprehensive, coordinated care using a payment model that holds organizations accountable for cost control and quality gains.

Change is already happening in the hospice landscape because value-based care models encompass all levels of care (from primary care to home health, long-term care, hospital, palliative care, and hospice) and force health care organizations to cooperate for better outcomes from diagnosis to the end of life (Exhibit 4.1). In 2021, the CMS added a hospice component to the Medicare Advantage Value-Based Insurance Design Model, commonly called the Medicare Advantage hospice carve-in. The initiative, formally named Primary Care First, includes a spectrum of models to support patients with serious illnesses from diagnosis through end of life. The program is designed to control costs, reduce avoidable hospitalization, and improve care coordination. Primary Care First was initially slated to roll out in January 2021, but leaders in the hospice community lobbied Congress for a 2-year delay. Regardless of the official start, hospice agencies and their community partners continue to take steps toward a value-based payment environment.

IMPLICATIONS FOR OCCUPATIONAL THERAPY

The current per-diem payment model in hospice and the larger movement toward interagency value-based care have real-world implications for occupational therapy practitioners. Currently, some hospice agencies may be reluctant to add services (i.e., request occupational therapy evaluations) that are considered supplemental to the Medicare-required services in hospice if they do not readily see the value in those services (e.g., a nurse and social worker are required for every hospice case, but occupational therapy is ordered as needed). Hospice agencies may be even more reluctant to spend limited resources on occupational therapy services if stakeholders believe therapy practitioners to be working counter to the hospice philosophy (i.e., some teammates may consider

EXHIBIT 4.1.

DEMONSTRATING OCCUPATIONAL THERAPY'S VALUE IN HOSPICE

Emerging value-based care models prioritize

- high-quality patient- and family-centered services (i.e., applying quality measures)
- effective coordination of care
- support for patients and families where they live
- timely transition to hospice to maximize the full benefit
- reduction in unnecessary hospitalizations and other resource-heavy care
- patient and family satisfaction.

Occupational therapy practitioners interested in or working in end-of-life care may reflect on key questions, including

- "Where does the money come from that ultimately supports my compensation?"
- "What is the payment system that provides that money? How does the provision of [occupational therapy] services fit into that payment system?"
- "Is there a value-based payment component?"
- "What does my position cost the agency (total compensation)?"
- "How does what I do contribute to quality, service, and cost as defined by this hospice?"
- "Are there any changes I may consider in my practice patterns that could potentially have a positive impact on quality, service, and/or cost measures for this hospice?"
- "Am I able to articulate to a wide range of stakeholders how what I do/what [occupational therapy] does contributes to value as defined in hospice?" (Siebert, 2022, slide 33).

occupational therapy to be aggressive treatment or are only familiar with a rehabilitative approach in therapy focused on remediating functional skills). For these reasons, occupational therapy practitioners remain underused in hospice (e.g., the hospice physician may request a single therapy evaluation, for example, to determine rehabilitation potential for a patient who is considering revoking hospice or to determine safe eating or feeding strategies for someone with dysphagia, but not for ongoing care). Occupational therapy could be used more routinely in the hospice setting, though, because it offers a rich opportunity to improve comfort and QoL for patients and families.

In advocating for occupational therapy in hospice, occupational therapy practitioners need to educate others that Medicare policy specifically names occupational therapy as a covered service within the Medicare hospice benefit. In addition to the hospice core services (physician services, nursing services, medical social services, and counseling), physical, occupational, and speech therapy services must be made available, under physician order, by all Medicare-certified hospice agencies to meet the needs of the patient and family (CMS, 2021a). This does not mean that every person who is receiving hospice care is appropriate for or will automatically receive occupational therapy services. However, it does signify that all Medicare beneficiaries who are receiving end-of-life care from a Medicare-certified hospice agency have the right to access occupational therapy services if there is a need for skilled help to control symptoms, manage pain, optimize basic functional skills, and maximize occupational participation as the disease progresses. Hospice agencies located in areas classified by the U.S. Census Bureau as nonurban may be granted a waiver by CMS if they are unable to access rehabilitation staff such as occupational therapy practitioners as the result of an inability to recruit appropriate personnel despite diligent efforts. Although full-time employee positions at hospice agencies remain limited for practitioners, there may be opportunities to develop partnerships with hospice agencies and possibly develop part-time positions or contracts to meet the agency's therapy needs.

Expanding occupational therapy's role in end-of-life care requires advocacy from diverse stakeholders, including hospice patients and their families who may advocate for occupational therapy, members of the interdisciplinary hospice team, and occupational therapy practitioners profession-wide. It is important to note that occupational therapy practitioners are already working with a vast population of people living with chronic disease across a wide range of nonhospice end-of-life care settings (e.g., home health agencies, acute care, and skilled nursing facilities; Chow et al., 2022b). Therefore, it behooves all practitioners to notice clinical signs indicating hospice eligibility, facilitate appropriate care transitions with effective communication and teamwork, and support occupational participation for patients nearing the end of life and their families, regardless of the practice setting (Chow et al., 2018). Occupational therapy practitioners working in a wide range of practice settings can be instrumental in helping patients access and receive their full hospice benefit at the right time if they

- stay aware of general hospice eligibility guidelines;
- recognize clinical and functional signs that a person could be nearing the end of life; and
- communicate with patients, families, and the interdisciplinary team about hospice

A common misconception is that occupational therapy is not covered in hospice. However, it is critical to note that Medicare policy guidelines do not exclude occupational therapy in the event of a terminal condition or election to receive palliative or hospice services. Specifically, the Medicare hospice benefit includes the provision of rehabilitative services in hospice care and states that for people receiving hospice services, "physical therapy, occupational therapy, and speech–language pathology services may be provided for purposes of symptom control or to enable the individual to maintain activities of daily living and basic functional skills" (CMS, 2021a, p. 33).

HOSPICE BENEFIT PERIODS

Hospice care is organized temporally into benefit periods. The first two periods are 90 days each, and each subsequent benefit period is 60 days. At the beginning of each period, the hospice medical director must write a summary of the patient, detailing why they continue to be eligible for hospice, and submit it to the patient's insurance for review. Hospice is also required to discuss every patient at an interdisciplinary team meeting, consisting of, at a minimum, the physician, nurse, social worker, and chaplain, every 2 weeks.

LEVELS OF HOSPICE CARE

There are four levels of hospice care. ***Routine care*** is the norm and makes up the vast majority of hospice days. Routine care may include pain and other symptom management, emotional and spiritual counseling for the patient and family; assistance with personal care; nutritional services; and therapy aimed at maximizing participation, comfort, and QoL. Routine hospice care is provided where the patient lives. The usual locations are homes, assisted living facilities, or nursing homes, but other places such as jails or homeless shelters are occasionally sites for routine hospice care. Routine care is provided intermittently on the basis of the needs of the patient and family. Additionally, hospice doctors and nurses are available 24 hours a day to answer questions or assist patients and families should sudden needs arise.

The second level is respite care. Medicare will pay for up to 5 nights at a time of respite care to allow caregivers a break or to allow for a location change. For example, if a patient at home is worsening to the point that their family can no longer safely care for them, they could be admitted to respite care while working on placement in a nursing home. Respite care is typically given in a hospice unit or a contracted bed in a hospital or nursing home.

General inpatient and continuous home care are the final levels of care, and they are reserved for patients who are having symptoms that cannot be adequately managed in routine care. Inpatient care is for treatment in an inpatient facility, either a hospice unit or a contracted bed in a hospital or nursing home; continuous home care deploys inpatient-type care at home, with the presence of hospice personnel in the home at least 8 hours per day.

INTERDISCIPLINARY HOSPICE TEAM

The Medicare hospice benefit stipulates that an interdisciplinary group work together for the holistic care of the hospice beneficiary. The core hospice team members are the nurse, physician, social worker, chaplain, bereavement specialist, home health aide, and hospice volunteer. Not all disciplines are involved with every patient, though. Hospice patients and families may choose to decline spiritual care, for example, or aide services if those needs are met by others in their inner circle. The Medicare hospice benefit includes supplemental services, such as occupational therapy, physical therapy, speech–language pathology, massage therapy, music therapy, art therapy, pet therapy, and dietary services. Hospice patients should have access to supplemental services, and those services can be added anytime to the plan of care because they are already covered by hospice. Although a minimum number of services are required to be performed by hospice employees (e.g., nursing, medical social work, counseling), supplemental services (e.g., occupational therapy, physician specialty services) may be contracted by the hospice to meet unusual staffing needs (CMS, 2021a).

The fluid nature of the hospice team (team members are continuously added or subtracted on the basis of the patient's and family's evolving needs) points to the importance of interprofessional communication and collaboration in daily practice to ensure the best outcomes for everyone involved (Mertens et al., 2019). For that reason, interprofessional education that includes nonclinical staff (i.e., nursing assistants, housekeepers, and clerical staff, among others, who are integral to the care process but historically excluded from interprofessional education) is recommended in this setting. For example, Broglio et al. (2019) found that interprofessional educational programs for blended hospice teams were effective in boosting team members' shared knowledge and team collaboration and significantly reduced emotional exhaustion and depersonalization. Such overall improvements in team function could potentially have additional positive impacts on patient outcomes and experiences with end-of-life care, so all hospice teammates are encouraged to remain ready for interprofessional learning on diverse teams.

Evidence Supporting the Effectiveness of Hospice

The literature contains good evidence that hospice accomplishes what it is intended to do: Improve QoL for patients and their families who are facing a life-limiting illness. The data show that hospice care results in better symptom management (Cheraghlou et al., 2016), lower rates of depression and complicated grief among the bereaved (Bradley et al., 2004), lower medical spending and rehospitalizations in the final months (Huo et al., 2014; Taylor et al., 2007), and overall improved satisfaction for family members (Schockett et al., 2005). Families consistently report feeling that they were referred to hospice too late (Rickerson et al., 2005; Teno et al., 2007). Indeed, the average length of stay in hospice is only 18 days (NHPCO, 2021), but the evidence shows that the longer a patient is in hospice, the more benefit they receive. It is not at all uncommon for a patient to die the same day they are referred to hospice. This short amount of time does not allow for patients and families to receive the full benefit of hospice services. Earlier enrollment, which hinges on a timely referral, allows patients and families to fully use the whole cadre of medical and support services included in the hospice benefit.

Occupational Therapy's Distinct Value in End-of-Life Care

Transitioning into hospice care can be one of the most critical and challenging life experiences for the person nearing the end of life and their loved ones. Occupational therapy's distinct value in end-of-life care is in enhancing QoL by facilitating occupation for the patient and their family during the patient's remaining time (American Occupational Therapy Association [AOTA], 2016). The need for occupational therapy often increases for these patients as they become simultaneously concerned with living and dying (Bye, 1998; Hasselkus & Jacques, 1998). For example, hospice patients typically experience significant losses in daily routines and separation from meaningful occupations as their disease progresses (Peoples et al., 2017). The resulting state of occupational deprivation has a significant negative impact on the person's perceived health and well-being (Keesing & Rosenwax, 2011; Yerxa, 1998). When valued occupational roles are disrupted, people can experience diminished self-identity, lack of daily structure, and social isolation (Ericksson et al., 2016). However, maintaining ***occupational participation***—continued engagement in new or different ways as the disease progresses—can lend a sense of pleasure and competence (Sviden et al., 2010).

Despite the hospice patient's declining health, continued participation (prioritized over performance), facilitated through a positive, supportive, and compassionate environment, helps facilitate QoL and well-being (Pizzi & Richards, 2017). Occupation can serve as a comforting diversion for hospice patients and families, distracting them from the illness and bringing their attention to positive relationships and the value of everyday tasks (Lala & Kinsella, 2011). For example, one hospice patient may derive a feeling of normalcy from doing his family's laundry. For this person, the importance of the activity was less about the task itself (his family would have happily done the laundry) and more about the positive feeling he gained from contributing to the household chores while he still could.

For some, the desire to continue living is closely linked to the ability to participate in enjoyable leisure activities (Lala & Kinsella, 2011). For example, a patient receives a terminal cancer diagnosis and suddenly loses many of her valued occupations. At first, she feels intense grief, but eventually her sadness shifts to boredom and anxiety; she describes herself as "waiting to die." Relief comes in the form of her favorite sister-in-law, who comes to town to do fun things in their remaining time together. The two ladies pass the next few months playing cards, making meals, watching funny movies, and laughing together as they have done for decades.

Achieving meaningful occupational experiences, solitary and shared, has been shown to facilitate gratitude and joy—making life worth living (Lyons et al., 2002). Occupation allows people at the end of life to adapt, cope, reflect, learn, live, do, appreciate, contribute, prioritize, and fulfill their potential during a special time of life (Benthall & Holmes, 2011). For many, occupation can make the difference between a good death experience and undue suffering for everyone involved. For all these reasons, participation in meaningful life occupations remains as important and health supporting in all environments at the end of life as it is in earlier stages (AOTA, 2016; Chow & Pickens, 2020; Jacques & Hasselkus, 2004).

Occupational therapy practitioners are the most qualified to address the occupational needs of patients who are close to death. With consideration of personal and multilevel contextual factors, practitioners facilitate participation through modification of occupations and the environment, compensatory strategies, caregiver training, and bereavement support (Hammill et al., 2014; Mills & Payne, 2015; Pickens, 2011). Research has suggested that practitioners working in this area integrate their understanding of the dying process with strategies to help dying patients continue to live meaningful lives (despite inevitable functional decline) while supporting them through physical, emotional, and existential loss and preparing them for death (Bye, 1998; Hammill et al., 2014; Hasselkus & Jacques, 1998).

Occupational therapy practitioners working in hospice are interested in the full range of their patients' chosen occupations and acknowledge that certain occupations may be reinterpreted or take on different significance as the person, family, or both prepares for the person's death (Jacques & Hasselkus, 2004; la Cour et al., 2009; Morgan, 2012). For example, continuing an ordinary activity such as eating dinner together while watching a favorite television program could strengthen feelings of connectedness for the person and family when they know that their time together is limited. An important family milestone (e.g., sharing a grandchild's birthday cake) may feel even more meaningful against the backdrop of the patient's end-of-life care (Jacques & Hasselkus, 2004). Occupations at the end of life are often dynamic and social as the person's illness progresses and more caregiver support is needed.

For example, a mother's desire to do things with her young children remains strong as her disease progresses, so she, her spouse, and the occupational therapist work together to continuously adjust how she experiences participation (not performance) with her children. Eventually, the woman is spending most of her time in bed, so her spouse facilitates the children playing in the same room, allowing the sights and sounds of their activity to surround her. Occupations at the end of life may be complex or mundane, but the near-death situation seems to heighten the meaning of occupational choices for the dying person and those around them (Jacques & Hasselkus, 2004). Of all the members of the hospice team, occupational therapy practitioners best understand the nature of occupation at this special time of life and occupation's role in creating meaningful, positive experiences, and they are therefore most equipped to identify and attend to the occupational needs of patients who are simultaneously living and dying (Benthall & Holmes, 2011).

Evidence Supporting Occupation's Benefits at End of Life

Although intervention research in the practice area of hospice still lags behind other occupational therapy research, the links among occupation, symptom relief, QoL, and a perceived good death provide some of the strongest support for expanding occupational therapy's role in hospice (Chow & Pickens, 2020). For example, research has shown that people living with a terminal illness still value being able to engage in daily self-care routines as long as possible (Eriksson et al., 2016; Peoples et al., 2017).

Toward the aim of maximizing occupational performance in the patient's remaining time, Lee et al.'s (2005) prospective study was the first to show that end-stage cancer patients could eat and drink more independently when occupational therapy took a compensatory approach and interventions included positioning, feeding aid support, and upper limb support. Kasven-Gonzalez et al. (2010) found that when occupational therapy addressed ADL retraining, functional transfer training, and family education, the patient's functional status improved temporarily during the last 7 weeks of terminal cancer. According to their case report, the occupational therapy intervention afforded the patient a greater sense of control and engagement in goal setting, and the outcomes were meaningful to the patient regardless of her limited life expectancy (Kasven-Gonzalez et al., 2010).

Norris (1999) assessed occupational performance and satisfaction in valued occupations using the Canadian Occupational Performance Measure before and after occupational therapy intervention with 18 participants in palliative care. After therapy that included self-care training, socialization, and leisure activities, 14 participants (78%) felt their performance improved, and 15 (83%) reported increased satisfaction (Norris, 1999). When inpatient oncology patients received occupational therapy focused on self-care retraining, functional transfers, household tasks, and energy conservation, they achieved 55% of their goals at or above expected levels using goal attainment scaling (GAS; Panchmatia & Urch, 2014). Participants expressed satisfaction with the goal-setting process and appreciation for the opportunity to express their concerns to an occupational therapist. Thus, Panchmatia and Urch (2014) concluded that GAS was useful for facilitating communication with patients in end-of-life care and may help therapists justify the need for therapy.

In all of these studies, the participant's functional gains were expected to be temporary and contributed more to the patient's quality of remaining time, which is why occupational therapy practitioners and other stakeholders need to look beyond rehabilitation potential when determining the need for occupational therapy in hospice (Chow & Pickens, 2020).

Although self-care remains important to many patients living with a terminal illness, it makes up only a fraction of what patients want and need to do during their remaining time (Chow & Pickens, 2020). Other studies have identified that patients nearing the end of life express new occupational concerns specific to the final stage of the life course. These desired ***end-of-life occupations*** include prioritizing relationships, reworking life to accommodate progressive illness, engaging in life review and legacy building, finding closure, putting affairs in order, and making final arrangements (Hunter, 2008; Jacques & Hasselkus, 2004; Lala & Kinsella, 2011).

In one study investigating an occupation-based programmatic intervention designed to teach life management skills to patients with a terminal illness, participants described a typical day and were educated on fatigue, energy levels, energy conservation, sleep, relaxation, and activity analysis and modification. After the program, most individuals (7 of 8) experienced better symptom management and less fatigue, and were better able to manage daily life during that time (Littlechild, 2016). Similarly, Miller and Hopkinson (2008) investigated a relaxation program consisting of written scripts, neuromuscular relaxation, autosuggestion, and visualization and found positive effects on patients' symptom of tension, presumably affording additional opportunities for meaningful occupational engagement.

Sakaguchi and Okamura (2015) took a creative, artistic approach to end-of-life occupation when they examined narratives of older adult patients with cancer using a life review collage activity. In the first session, the occupational therapist conducted a life review interview with the patient and facilitated the patient in collecting collage images. In the second and final session, the therapist and patient created the collage booklet together, based on the interview. The artistic occupation was an effective modality to support spiritual well-being and self-efficacy; address anxiety and depression; and facilitate end-of-life conversations among patients, family, and staff in palliative care inpatient settings (Sakaguchi & Okamura, 2015).

Yamaga et al. (2021) described a clinical case of a patient with end-stage prostate cancer whose occupational therapy focused on participation in the patient's most meaningful occupation: playing music. Before becoming ill, the patient had worked and played music as a hobby; he organized live concerts, played the guitar, and composed music. As the patient's cancer metastasized to other areas of his body and a pathological fracture of the left humerus was causing significant pain, he spent most of his time alone in the hospital room, confined to the bed. The patient expressed his main concerns: "I want to play music, but I cannot do it because I cannot move left arm. There is no hope of living now." The purpose of occupational therapy for this patient was to enable him to participate in his chosen occupation for the rest of his life; guided by the occupational therapist, the patient set a goal to play a concert at the hospital. During the course of his occupational therapy, the patient relearned to play the guitar, gathered band members, and prepared for the concert. Throughout the intervention period, the therapist helped the patient manage pain and improve function in his left arm to play the guitar. During occupational therapy sessions, the patient made posters to recruit band members from among the medical staff who played musical instruments and wrote music for the concert. Between occupational therapy sessions, the band practiced. The patient's roles and routines in the occupation were similar to those he enacted before his hospitalization. As a result of the month-long intervention, the patient was able to participate in his most preferred musical activities; he was no longer confined to his hospital room, his QoL improved from baseline, and his anxiety and depression decreased. Just before the concert, 105 days postintervention, the patient developed respiratory symptoms due to a metastatic lung tumor and subsequently died. However, the occupational therapy intervention supported the patient in participating in his most meaningful occupation, even at the end of life, enabling him to live each day to the fullest and maximize his QoL during his remaining time (Yamaga et al., 2021).

Perhaps the best demonstration of occupation's benefits at the end of life is seen in qualitative research that describes ways in which occupational therapy may promote what terminally ill patients and families regard as a ***good death***. Researchers have summarized what a good death means from the terminally ill patient's perspective: a phenomenon including pain and symptom management, preparation for death, a sense of completion, feeling in control, being treated as a whole person, being as mentally aware or unaware as they wish, having affairs in order, not being a burden, being at peace spiritually, and helping others (Jacques & Hasselkus, 2004; Lyons et al., 2002; Singer et al., 1999; Steinhauser et al., 2000). Other research has suggested that patients and families would like to avoid a bad death, which they characterize as missing opportunities to plan, arrange personal affairs, decrease family burdens, or say goodbye (Steinhauser et al., 2000). Moreover, a good death is about what each person perceives as good, a unique experience for each dying person and their family (Jacques & Hasselkus, 2004).

Jacques and Hasselkus's (2004) qualitative study suggested new ways of thinking about occupation at the end of life and thereby invites more opportunities for occupational therapy practitioners to work with patients close to death. In their observations of hospice patients, occupation was how dying patients could continue living by choosing to do the things that really mattered to them. Occupation served as a mechanism to prepare for death, taking the form of completion activities that helped the person say goodbye to loved ones, share life stories, discuss end-of-life choices, give away personal items, or finalize funeral arrangements.

Occupation also eased the patients' and families' experience of waiting for death and the family's experience immediately after the death (Jacques & Hasselkus, 2004). The expanded perspective on the special nature of occupation at the end of life and its power to improve the death experience for all involved in the dying process reveals a greater need for occupational therapy—and a wider range of potential services provided by occupational therapy practitioners—to enable occupation in end-of-life care environments. As more stakeholders appreciate the ongoing significance of occupation in maintaining and shaping the last chapter of life and understand occupational therapy's full supportive role as it aligns with the hospice philosophy, more hospice patients may continue living with purpose, as proactive occupational beings throughout the last stage of their illness (Chow et al., 2022a; Lyons et al., 2002; see Case Example 4.3).

Some may mistakenly think that once a person chooses hospice care, there is no turning back. In fact, once enrolled in hospice care, patients are free to leave a hospice program at any time for any reason without penalty. Reenrollment in a hospice program is possible as long as the medical eligibility criteria are met. In addition, some patients could experience improvement in their overall health and no longer be eligible for hospice. Whether the bounce-back is temporary or long term, there is no limit to the number of times a person may receive their hospice benefit as long as they meet eligibility guidelines (HFA, 2018a).

Barriers to and Opportunities for Occupational Therapy Use

SERVICE GAP

Despite the health benefits of continued occupational participation, regardless of declining functional status, for terminally ill patients (Sviden et al., 2010) and occupational therapy's vital role in facilitating occupational participation for these patients and their families (AOTA, 2016; Yeh & McColl, 2019), occupational therapy practitioners remain underused in hospice care (Chow et al., 2022b; Knecht-Sabres et al., 2018; Mills & Payne, 2015). Experts acknowledge multiple extrinsic barriers contributing to low utilization, including insufficient reimbursement, limited employment opportunities, misunderstanding of occupational therapy's role, and insufficient research on the use of occupation-based interventions (Eva & Morgan, 2018; Keesing & Rosenwax, 2011; Knecht-Sabres et al., 2018). In addition, some practitioners may feel inadequately trained or

CASE EXAMPLE 4.3. SARA: PART 3

Sara's daughter reported that the decision to transition Sara home with hospice was among the best and most important decisions their family ever made. The occupational therapist working for hospice was instrumental in adapting activities, modifying the environment, and training caregivers to enable Sara to participate in meaningful occupations with her family. As the weeks passed and Sara's performance skills waned, she received more personal care assistance from caregivers so that she could preserve energy for her favorite activities with her grandson. Simple, everyday occupations such as teaching him to bake cookies, watching him play, and tucking him into bed at night took on new meaning for Sara and the family as they focused on making the most of their time together. Sara felt satisfied that she was there engaging with her daughter and grandson, even when she was too weak to perform tasks herself. Reading stories to the boy was something that Sara and he enjoyed equally. Knowing that her shortness of breath and fatigue would inevitably worsen, Sara and the therapist had an idea to make story time last longer. With help from the therapist, Sara chose some favorite children's books and recorded herself reading and speaking personal messages to the child while she still could. When reading was no longer possible, Sara and her grandson found it soothing and restful to listen to the recordings together.

Sara passed away 5 months after returning home. After her death, Sara's daughter expressed gratitude for the creative, occupation-based, and person- and family-centered care provided by the occupational therapist: "During the last months of Mom's life, she and my son were happiest curled up with their favorite stories. Without the support from occupational therapy, that most meaningful activity would have been lost sooner. And to think, we had story time all together even on Mom's last day. Mom's recordings are a lasting gift to us. As my son and I still listen together, we share memories of Mom and feel close to her still. Thank you for making it all possible."

underprepared for end-of-life care, posing an intrinsic barrier to utilization (Chow et al., 2022a; Eva & Morgan, 2018; Talbot-Coulombe & Guay, 2020). In the face of these real-world challenges, occupational therapy practitioners remain the profession's best advocates, so in this final section, we offer a few strategies to advance occupational therapy's utilization in this practice area.

ADVOCATING UPSTREAM TO CONNECT PATIENTS WITH THEIR FULL HOSPICE BENEFIT

Occupational therapy practitioners working with patients with serious illnesses in any practice setting can play a valuable role in helping patients maximize their hospice benefit as soon as the patient is eligible and ready by sharing general information about hospice in goals-of-care conversations and advanced care planning. A practitioner working in the hospital, rehabilitation facility, or long-term-care home may be the best conversation partner for patients and families who are thinking about their future in light of a progressive incurable disease and decline in the level of function.

Occupational therapy practitioners are trained in the therapeutic use of self, motivational interviewing techniques, and goal attainment and are therefore well equipped to help patients and families identify for themselves what is most important and the steps needed to achieve their end-of-life wishes. Practitioners spend time with patients and their families in intimate contexts, doing everyday activities, which affords opportunities for caring conversations about the patient's hopes for the future, their most valued roles and routines, and how they envision optimal participation in the event of decreasing functional capacities—time that is often unavailable to other providers. By framing the patient's challenges with a life-course perspective, practitioners can help patients and families understand the current problems they want to resolve, anticipate future challenges, and clarify for themselves what constitutes a good final chapter for their life, including whether, when, where, and with whom hospice fits in their plan. In these preliminary and proactive conversations about making the most of life all the way to the end, practitioners working upstream of hospice can support patients and families in exercising control by facilitating open discussions about death as a natural part of life; educating patients on care options, including palliative care and hospice; and encouraging patients to engage the important people in their life in the process (Jacques & Hasselkus, 2004).

Occupational therapy practitioners already working in end-of-life care have additional opportunities beyond direct patient care. Many hospice agencies are thinking proactively about steering those upstream care planning discussions themselves with a wider pool of providers in different settings to improve quality and timely access to goal-concordant care

(Vossel, 2021). The hospice's need for community liaisons to target care coordination presents an opportunity for occupational therapy practitioners inside the organization to advocate that they are well equipped for those goals-of-care conversations and a perfect partner to ease the burden of transition to hospice that exists for so many.

When it comes to addressing goals of care, occupational therapy practitioners bring a valuable occupational perspective of health, with expertise in advanced care planning discussions and documentation processes. An occupational therapy practitioner may be more successful at completing advanced care planning documents than others on the health care team because the practitioner centers the conversation around what the patient and family want and need to do during this time while collaboratively considering contextual factors, available supports, potential challenges, and creative solutions that fit the patient's situation. When practitioners notice and understand the challenges that their hospice agency is looking to solve, they can lean into opportunities to serve in other roles in addition to direct patient care (e.g., community liaison, consultant, occupation-based program developer).

DISPELLING MYTHS ABOUT OCCUPATIONAL THERAPY AND HOSPICE

It is a common misconception that occupational therapy services are either not appropriate for or not afforded to patients living with a terminal illness when, in fact, Medicare policy includes occupational therapy in hospice care as a covered and reimbursed service in all Medicare-certified agencies (Benthall & Holmes, 2011; CMS, 2021a). Occupational therapy practitioners working in any practice setting can reassure patients that electing their hospice benefit does not automatically mean discontinuing occupational therapy. Eligible patients might be more accepting of hospice if they know that occupational therapy is included in the Medicare hospice benefit to control symptoms, maintain functional skills that would otherwise be lost sooner, and enable the person to remain engaged in personally meaningful daily activities with progressive modifications for enhanced QoL (CMS, 2021a).

Families might also feel more supported and confident about transitioning their loved one to hospice if they know that occupational therapy services covered by the dying person's hospice benefit include caregiver training and support for everyone involved in the dying process, before, during, and after the loved one's death. In these situations, families may benefit from self-advocacy strategies to be able to articulate their desire and goals for occupational therapy that are consistent with the goals of hospice care.

SHIFTING OCCUPATIONAL THERAPY'S FOCUS IN END-OF-LIFE CARE TO FOREGROUND OCCUPATIONAL PARTICIPATION

Providing occupational therapy for patients receiving hospice care means aligning the goals of therapy with the hospice philosophy. This includes providing services to patients and caregivers that maximize comfort and QoL at the end of life, not curing illness. Thus, occupational therapy from a rehabilitative approach (aimed at restoring the patient's previous level of independence or progressively improving functional skills) does not fit with a hospice plan of care. Although occupational engagement remains essential and health supporting at the end of life, capturing the occupational needs of hospice patients requires a perspective shift. Once the aim of therapy shifts from a restorative or rehabilitative approach to one focused on enabling occupation for a good death, then occupational therapy practitioners may serve as vital partners with hospice patients and teammates in achieving end-of-life goals together and thereby bolster the use of occupational therapy.

We acknowledge that shifting occupational therapy practitioners' focus may sometimes feel easier said than done. Entering end-of-life care might feel challenging, even daunting for some practitioners, especially if the practitioner's prior training and work experiences prioritized increasing independence and improving functional skills for their patients. Practitioners may wonder, "How can I hop out of the rehab rut and harness the power of occupation with patients whose functional capacities are expected to decline?" Just like a subtle twist of a camera lens brings new things into focus while sending other things to the background, a subtle change in the practitioner's perspective can foreground what matters most in end-of-life care. For example, choosing to focus on occupational participation instead of isolated performance skills is a good first step that leads to more creative problem solving with hospice patients, families, and teammates. Ideas for adaptive compensatory strategies, activity modifications, environmental interventions, and caregiver training come into clearer view when the practitioner prioritizes participation over performance. When such participation-focused interventions are implemented together, the dying person may continue to have meaningful occupational experiences regardless of declining functional skills.

In addition to swapping performance for participation, practitioners can continue honing their practice with this population by embracing the concept of living while dying, acknowledging the evolving significance of occupation for the dying person and their family, and taking advantage of the full range of opportunities to enable occupation in various end-of-life care settings. As Bye (1998) noted,

> The outcome is not about independence or permanent rehabilitation to normal life—hallmarks of traditional occupational therapy. It is about occupational therapists helping clients to realize their goals to connect with life, and people in their life, on a level beyond illness and receipt of care. The achievement of this outcome affirms clients' lives. (p. 19)

Of course, any such shift toward occupation-based practice calls for more research. As Chow and Pickens (2020) noted in their review of the literature, the underutilization of occupational therapy in hospice may be attributable to a lack of evidence on efficacy. Therefore, more research is needed on interventions aptly focused on terminally ill patients' participation in end-of-life occupations and environmental influences on occupational engagement for them and their families.

COMMUNICATING OCCUPATIONAL THERAPY'S DISTINCT VALUE MORE EXPLICITLY FOR STAKEHOLDERS

Hospice patients and their families face a host of occupational challenges, yet relatively few patients are connected with occupational therapy during their time in hospice. One study found that only about 10% of a national sample of patients receiving hospice at home received occupational therapy as part of their hospice benefit (Mueller et al., 2021). The majority of the sample was expected to live at least 6 months after admission, suggesting that patients and families had time to consider the quality of their remaining time and how it might be enriched through participation in meaningful occupations, but missed the opportunity to do so with an occupational therapy practitioner. In that study, more than 87%

of the participants required assistance with at least one ADL, but fewer than 10% received support from occupational therapy to address ADLs, which suggests more missed opportunities for the use of occupational therapy. Moreover, patients who did not receive occupational therapy were 7 times more likely than those who did to use emergency care (11.5% vs. 1.7%, respectively). In their cases, emergency care included medication problems or complications; injury resulting from fall; wound infection, new lesion, or ulcer; and diabetes control issues, hypoglycemia, and hyperglycemia, among other urgent concerns that occupational therapy could help to avoid.

Ultimately, greater use of occupational therapy in hospice depends on more occupational therapy referrals—which requires that interdisciplinary team members know what occupational therapy practitioners do and their impact. In their study of occupational therapy utilization (i.e., adding occupational therapy to the hospice plan of care), Chow et al. (2022a) found that it was driven mostly by the decision makers' awareness of occupational therapy's role in end-of-life care and influenced by the demands of the setting and the decision makers' ability to see the purpose of the occupational therapy referral as addressing the patient's and/or family's QoL goals and the dying process.

Unfortunately, many decision makers lacked understanding of how functional loss can erode a person's autonomy, lead to occupational deprivation, and cause existential suffering. Additionally, decision makers lacked understanding of how occupational therapy practitioners could provide comfort through supported participation in daily activities. In addition to misunderstanding occupational therapy's intent in this practice area, some decision makers erroneously presumed occupational therapy is not reimbursed under the Medicare hospice benefit—usually because they viewed therapy as strictly rehabilitative. For hospice patients to gain improved occupational participation and patient or caregiver care experiences, decision makers must adjust their focus on what's available, meaningful, and valuable through occupational therapy in end-of-life care to improve QoL (Chow et al., 2022a).

More hospice teammates need to know the full scope of occupational therapy practice in end-of-life care to make appropriate and timely referrals for the service (Chow & Pickens, 2020; Chow et al., 2022a). It can be helpful for students and practitioners to connect their community partners with AOTA's official documents (AOTA, 2016) and talk more explicitly about occupational therapy's role in this practice area (see Exhibit 4.2):

- Occupational therapy practitioners' distinct value in end-of-life care is to facilitate QoL for patients and their caregivers through engagement in occupations during the patient's remaining days.
- Occupational therapy practitioners honor a person's full life course and believe that participation in meaningful occupations remains as important at the end of life as it is in the earlier stages.
- Occupational therapy practitioners working in end-of-life care intentionally align their practice with the hospice philosophy. Practitioners collaborate with the patient and family members throughout the occupational therapy process to identify occupations that are especially meaningful and incorporate strategies that support participation and QoL rather than rehabilitation.
- With support from occupational therapy practitioners, hospice patients and families can adapt and remain engaged in familiar, comforting roles and routines and explore new occupations that emerge as most meaningful when people are aware that they are close to the end of life.
- On the basis of evidence from research, occupational therapy practitioners understand the health-supporting nature of occupational participation for people living with a terminal illness and their families in helping them to achieve greater comfort, dignity, autonomy, and peace throughout the progression of the disease. Thus, practitioners facilitate a good death experience for everyone involved in the dying process by enabling occupation (AOTA, 2016).

EXHIBIT 4.2.

PROMOTING OCCUPATIONAL THERAPY IN END-OF-LIFE CARE

Occupational therapy practitioners may view and compare publicly reported quality measures for any hospice agency (or any other health care provider, for that matter) in their area at Care Compare on Medicare.gov (www.medicare.gov/care-compare). This site was created to help consumers compare hospice providers' performance and assist consumers in choosing the provider who is right for them. As such, the data serve as a useful reference for occupational therapy

(Continued)

EXHIBIT 4.2.
PROMOTING OCCUPATIONAL THERAPY IN END-OF-LIFE CARE *(Cont.)*

practitioners who want to explain how their services may help maintain or improve specific performance ratings that are most important to that hospice agency.

Many opportunities exist for occupational therapy practitioners to highlight their distinct value by understanding and applying quality measures to everyday practice (American Occupational Therapy Association, 2022). Whether it is a job interview, performance evaluation, routine documentation, or spontaneous conversation with a hospice patient, teammate, or community partner, all are opportunities for practitioners to connect the dots among occupational participation, quality of life (QoL), hospice philosophy, and the agency's value-based goals.

How Can You Promote Occupational Therapy's Value in End-of-Life Care?

- Keep up to date with policy and payment changes related to hospice and value-based care models.
- Look for opportunities to demonstrate the positive health effects of continued occupational participation at the end of life, despite the patient's expected performance decline.
- Identify and address patients' occupational concerns as they relate to new end-of-life occupations as well as familiar preferred roles and routines.
- Focus on evidence-based practice specific to occupational therapy at the end of life (not traditional rehabilitative models and not duplicative services).
- Be patient and family focused throughout the dying process and bereavement period.
- Focus on quality care and outcomes that align with the hospice philosophy, especially QoL, well-being, and satisfaction for the patient and family.
- Document services, explicitly relating the patient's and family's occupational concerns; the occupational therapy intervention; enhanced participation; and QoL, well-being, and satisfaction.
- Make value your product (e.g., share with people that occupational therapy is included in the Medicare hospice benefit and is a covered service for all hospice patients; know the publicly shared quality measures in hospice; explain how occupational therapy practitioners provide direct patient care and programmatic interventions to positively affect quality, efficiency, and satisfaction in end-of-life care).
- Advocate for yourself, your patients, and occupational therapy in language relevant to the stakeholder (i.e., patient, coworker, manager, administrator, payer, policymaker, public).

Summary

In light of all the opportunities and challenges in this rewarding practice area, we remain optimistic that occupational therapy will enjoy greater utilization and interdisciplinary support in end-of-life care in the future as the profession itself represents the change we want to see. We believe that the need for the paradigm shift (dropping rehabilitative models, picking up QoL via occupational participation), corresponding ways of practice and research, and communication with diverse stakeholders starts with us. Throughout this chapter, we have described a lot about occupational therapy and hospice, including who does what, when, where, and why. We have even suggested some advocacy steps that any practitioner or student could take to advance occupational therapy in hospice.

Heather McKay, PhD, OTR/L, is an occupational therapist, dementia care specialist, and international trainer and speaker on topics related to dementia care and caregiver education. She has over 20 years of experience working with older adults and their myriad caregivers across various settings. Currently, she is the founder and manager of Partnerships for Health, a dementia consulting company providing education and support for professionals and families and consultation with organizations on dementia workforce development. In addition to her work in dementia care education, Heather enjoys teaching in the Division of Occupational Science and Occupational Therapy at the University of North Carolina at Chapel Hill where she shares her experience and scholarship around productive aging, collective occupational adaptation, and occupational therapy in end-of-life care.

Christian H. Jacobus, MD, FACEP, FAAHPM, is the Hospice Medical Director for Bridge Home Health and Hospice in Findlay, Ohio. He is board certified in both emergency medicine and hospice and palliative medicine. He loves his clinical practice but is also passionate about teaching, especially on the intersection of palliative care and the emergency department.

David Benthall, MS, OTR/L, is an occupational therapist with a passion for serving older adult clients and caregivers in their homes and communities. David is currently working in Home Based Primary Care at the Durham VA Medical Center. He has previously worked in home health and hospice care settings and has served as an adjunct faculty member at the University of North Carolina at Chapel Hill's Division of Occupational Science and Occupational Therapy. David has presented and published on the topic of occupational therapy in end-of-life care and advocacy in primary health care.

REFERENCES

Almack, K., Cox, K., Moghaddam, N., Pollock, K., & Seymour, J. (2012). After you: Conversations between patients and healthcare professionals in planning for end-of-life care. *BMC Palliative Care, 11*(1), 15–15. https://doi.org/10.1186/1472-684X-11-15

American Cancer Society. (2019, May). *What is hospice care?* https://www.cancer.org/treatment/end-of-life-care/hospice-care/what-is-hospice-care.html

American Occupational Therapy Association. (2016). The role of occupational therapy in end-of-life care. *American Journal of Occupational Therapy, 70*(Suppl. 2), 7012410075. https://doi.org/10.5014/ajot.2016.706S17

American Occupational Therapy Association. (2022). *Quality: Volume to value—Providing high-value occupational therapy.* https://www.aota.org/practice/practice-essentials/quality/volume-to-value

Anderson, F., Downing, G. M., & Hill, J. (1996). Palliative Performance Scale (PPS): A new tool. *Journal of Palliative Care, 12*(1), 5–11. https://doi.org/10.1177/082585979601200102

Baxter, R., Fromme, E. K., & Sandgren, A. (2022). Patient identification for serious illness conversations: A scoping review. *International Journal of Environmental Research and Public Health, 19,* 4162. https://doi.org/10.3390/ijerph19074162

Benthall, D., & Holmes, T. (2011). End-of-life care: Facilitating meaningful occupations. *OT Practice, 16*(9), 7–10.

Bradley, E. H., Prigerson, H., Carlson, M. D. A., Cherlin, E., Johnson-Hurzeler, R., & Kasl, S. V. (2004). Depression among surviving caregivers: Does length of hospice enrollment matter? *American Journal of Psychiatry, 161,* 2257–2262. https://doi.org/10.1176/appi.ajp.161.12.2257

Brighton, L. J., & Bristowe, K. (2016). Communication in palliative care: Talking about the end of life, before the end of life. *Postgraduate Medical Journal, 92,* 466–470. https://doi.org/10.1136/postgradmedj-2015-133368

Broderick, A. (2020, January 29). *Veterans Affairs moves the needle in median LOS with concurrent care hospice.* Center to Advance Palliative Care. https://www.capc.org/blog/veterans-affairs-moves-needle-median-los-concurrent-care-hospice/

Broglio, K., DiMilia, P., Miller, J., Thomson, R., Garland, M., & Bruce, M. (2019). The gang's all here: All-inclusive interprofessional education in a palliative and hospice center (S809). *Journal of Pain and Symptom Management, 57,* 485–485. https://doi.org/10.1016/j.jpainsymman.2018.12.262

Bye, R. A. (1998). When clients are dying: Occupational therapists' perspectives. *Occupational Therapy Journal of Research, 18,* 3–24. https://doi.org/10.1177/153944929801800101

Cagle, J. G., Lee, J., Ornstein, K. A., & Guralnik, J. M. (2020). Hospice utilization in the United States: A prospective cohort study comparing cancer and noncancer deaths. *Journal of the American Geriatrics Society, 68,* 783–793. https://doi.org/10.1111/jgs.16294

Centers for Disease Control and Prevention. (2022). *About chronic diseases.* https://www.cdc.gov/chronicdisease/about/index.htm

Centers for Medicare & Medicaid Services. (2021a). Coverage of hospice services under hospital insurance. In *Medicare benefit policy manual* (Rev. 11056). https://www.cms.gov/manuals/Downloads/bp102c09.pdf

Centers for Medicare & Medicaid Services. (2021b). *Hospice determining terminal status.* https://www.cms.gov/medicare-coverage-database/view/lcd.aspx?LCDId=34538

Centers for Medicare and Medicaid Services. (2022a). *Hospice.* https://www.cms.gov/Medicare/Medicare-Fee-for-Service-Payment/Hospice

Centers for Medicare & Medicaid Services. (2022b). *Medicare Care Choices Model: Findings at a glance.* https://innovation.cms.gov/innovation-models/medicare-care-choices

Cheraghlou, S., Gahbauer, E. A., Leo-Summers, L., Stabenau, H. F., Chaudhry, S. I., & Gill, T. M. (2016). Restricting symptoms before and after admission to hospice. *American Journal of Medicine, 129,* 754.e7–754.e15. https://doi.org/10.1016/j.amjmed.2016.02.017

Chow, J. K., McKay, M. H., & Pickens, N. D. (2018). Management of end-of-life issues. In R. J. Gatchel, I. Z. Schultz, & C. T. Ray (Eds.), *Handbook of rehabilitation in older adults* (pp. 461–477). Springer. https://doi.org/10.1007/978-3-030-03916-5_24

Chow, J. K., & Pickens, N. D. (2020). Measuring the efficacy of occupational therapy in end-of-life care: A scoping review. *American Journal of Occupational Therapy, 74,* 7401205020. https://doi.org/10.5014/ajot.2020.033340

Chow, J. K., Pickens, N. D., Fletcher, T., Bowyer, P., & Thompson, M. (2022a). Missed opportunities to ease suffering: An explanatory model of occupational therapy utilization in end-of-life care. *American Journal of Hospice & Palliative Medicine,* 104990912211439-10499091221143917. doi:10.1177/10499091221143917

Chow, J. K., Pickens, N. D., Fletcher, T., Thompson, M., & Bowyer, P. (2022b). "You've got to do something": Developing occupational therapists' role in end-of-life care. *OTJR: Occupation, Participation and Health, 43,* 109–118. https://doi.org/10.1177/15394492221088239

Clayton, J. M., Hancock, K., Parker, S., Butow, P. N., Walder, S., Carrick, S., . . . Tattersall, M. H. N. (2008). Sustaining hope when communicating with terminally ill patients and their families: A systematic review. *Psycho-Oncology, 17,* 641–659. https://doi.org/10.1002/pon.1288

Eriksson, L., Oster, I., & Lindberg, M. (2016). The meaning of occupation for patients in palliative care when in hospital. *Palliative and Supportive Care, 14,* 541–552. https://doi.org/10.1017/S1478951515001352

Eva, G., & Morgan, D. (2018). Mapping the scope of occupational therapy practice in palliative care: A European Association for Palliative Care cross-sectional survey. *Palliative Medicine, 32*, 960–968. https://doi.org/10.1177/0269216318758928

Foerster, R. (2020, April 28). *How the Quadruple Aim and value-based care intersect.* Privia Health. https://www.priviahealth.com/blog/how-the-quadruple-aim-and-value-based-care-intersect/

Hammill, K., Bye, R., & Cook, C. (2014). Occupational therapy for people living with a life-limiting illness: A thematic review. *British Journal of Occupational Therapy, 77*, 582–589. https://doi.org/10.4276/030802214X14151078348594

Hasselkus, B. R., & Jacques, N. D. (1998). Occupational therapy and hospice. *American Journal of Occupational Therapy, 52*, 872–873.

Hospice Foundation of America. (2018a). *Dispelling hospice myths.* https://hospicefoundation.org/End-of-Life-Support-and-Resources/Coping-with-Terminal-Illness/Dispelling-Hospice-Myths

Hospice Foundation of America. (2018b). *What is hospice?* https://hospicefoundation.org/Hospice-Care/Hospice-Services

Hunter, E. G. (2008). Legacy: The occupational transmission of self through actions and artifacts. *Journal of Occupational Science, 15*, 48–54. https://doi.org/10.1080/14427591.2008.9686607

Huo, J., Lairson, D. R., Du, X. L., Chan, W., Buchholz, T. A., & Guadagnolo, B. A. (2014). Survival and cost-effectiveness of hospice care for metastatic melanoma patients. *American Journal of Managed Care, 20*, 366–373. https://www.ajmc.com/view/survival-and-cost-effectiveness-of-hospice-care-for-metastatic-melanoma-patients

Jacques, N. D., & Hasselkus, B. R. (2004). The nature of occupation surrounding dying and death. *OTJR: Occupation, Participation and Health, 24*, 44–53. https://doi.org/10.1177/153944920402400202

Karnofsky, D. A., & Burchenal, J. H. (1949). The clinical evaluation of chemotherapeutic agents in cancer. In C. M. MacLeod (Ed.), *Evaluation of chemotherapeutic agents* (pp. 191–205). Columbia University Press.

Kasven-Gonzalez, N., Souverain, R., & Miale, S. (2010). Improving quality of life through rehabilitation in palliative care: Case report. *Palliative and Supportive Care, 8*, 359–369. https://doi.org/10.1017/S1478951510000167

Keesing, S., & Rosenwax, L. (2011). Is occupation missing from occupational therapy in palliative care? *Australian Occupational Therapy Journal, 58*, 329–336. https://doi.org/10.1111/j.1440-1630.2011.00958.x

Knecht-Sabres, L. J., Weppner, A., Powers, C., & Siesel, B. (2018). Do health-care professionals really understand the role of occupational therapy in hospice care? *American Journal of Hospice and Palliative Medicine, 36*, 379–386. https://doi.org/10.1177/1049909118812858

Kumar, P., Wright, A. A., Hatfield, L. A., Temel, J. S., & Keating, N. L. (2017). Family perspectives on hospice care experiences of patients with cancer. *Journal of Clinical Oncology, 35,* 432–439. https://doi.org/10.1200/JCO.2016.68.9257

la Cour, K., Johannessen, H., & Josephsson, S. (2009). Activity and meaning making in the everyday lives of people with advanced cancer. *Palliative and Supportive Care, 7,* 469–479. https://doi.org/10.1017/S1478951509990472

Lala, A. P., & Kinsella, E. A. (2011). A phenomenological inquiry into the embodied nature of occupation at end of life. *Canadian Journal of Occupational Therapy, 78,* 246–254. https://doi.org/10.2182/cjot.2011.78.4.6

LaPointe, J. (2022, March 2). What is value-based care, what it means for providers? *Recycle Intelligence.* https://revcycleintelligence.com/features/what-is-value-based-care-what-it-means-for-providers

Lee, W. T. K., Chan, H. F., & Wong, E. (2005). Improvement of feeding independence in end-stage cancer patients under palliative care—A prospective, uncontrolled study. *Supportive Care in Cancer, 13,* 1051–1056. https://doi.org/10.1007/s00520-005-0859-7

Lindley, L. C., Keim-Malpass, J., Svynarenko, R., Cozad, M. J., Mack, J. W., & Hinds, P. S. (2020). Pediatric concurrent hospice care: A scoping review and directions for future nursing research. *Journal of Hospice and Palliative Nursing, 22,* 238–245. https://doi.org/10.1097/NJH.0000000000000648

Littlechild, B. (2016). Managing fatigue: A trial of group and individual educational support for hospice outpatients. *European Journal of Palliative Care, 23,* 166–168.

Lyons, M., Orozovic, N., Davis, J., & Newman, J. (2002). Doing–being–becoming: Occupational experiences of persons with life-threatening illnesses. *American Journal of Occupational Therapy, 56,* 285–295. https://doi.org/10.5014/ajot.56.3.285

McCaffrey, N., Bradley, S., Ratcliffe, J., & Currow, D. C. (2016). What aspects of quality of life are important from palliative care patients' perspectives? A systematic review of qualitative research. *Journal of Pain and Symptom Management, 52*(2), 318–328. https://doi.org/10.1016/j.jpainsymman.2016.02.012

Medicare Payment Advisory Commission. (2021). *March 2021 report to the Congress: Medicare payment policy.* https://www.medpac.gov/document/march-2021-report-to-the-congress-medicare-payment-policy/

Mertens, F., De Gendt, A., Deveugele, M., Van Hecke, A., & Pype, P. (2019). Interprofessional collaboration within fluid teams: Community nurses' experiences with palliative home care. *Journal of Clinical Nursing, 28,* 3680–3690. https://doi.org/10.1111/jocn.14969

Miller, J., & Hopkinson, C. (2008). A retrospective audit exploring the use of relaxation as an intervention in oncology and palliative care. *European Journal of Cancer Care, 17,* 488–491. https://doi.org/10.1111/j.1365-2354.2007.00899.x

Mills, K., & Payne, A. (2015). Enabling occupation at the end of life: A literature review. *Palliative and Supportive Care, 13,* 1755–1769. https://doi.org/10.1017/S1478951515000772

Mor, V., Wagner, T. H., Levy, C., Ersek, M., Miller, S. C., Gidwani-Marszowksi, R., . . . Shreve, S. (2019). Association of expanded VA hospice care with aggressive care and cost for veterans with advanced lung cancer. *JAMA Oncology, 5,* 810–816. https://doi.org/10.1001/jamaoncol.2019.0081

Morgan, D. D. (2012). *The ordinary becomes extraordinary: The occupation of living whilst dying* [Unpublished doctoral thesis]. University of Melbourne, Dentistry and Health Sciences, Faculty of Medicine, School of Health Sciences. http://hdl.handle.net/11343/37059

Mueller, E., Arthur, P., Ivy, M., Pryor, L., Armstead, A., & Li, C. (2021). Addressing the gap: Occupational therapy in hospice care. *Occupational Therapy in Health Care, 35,* 125–137. https://doi.org/10.1080/07380577.2021.1879410

Mulville, A. K., Widick, N. N., & Makani, N. S. (2019). Timely referral to hospice care for oncology patients: A retrospective review. *American Journal of Hospice and Palliative Care, 36,* 466–471. https://doi.org/10.1177/1049909118820494

National Hospice and Palliative Care Organization. (2018). *Standards of practice for hospice programs.* https://www.nhpco.org/wp-content/uploads/2019/04/Standards_Hospice_2018.pdf

National Hospice and Palliative Care Organization. (2020). *NHPCO facts and figures.* https://www.nhpco.org/wp-content/uploads/NHPCO-Facts-Figures-2020-edition.pdf

National Hospice and Palliative Care Organization. (2021). *NHPCO facts and figures.* https://www.nhpco.org/wp-content/uploads/NHPCO-Facts-Figures-2021.pdf

National Hospice and Palliative Care Organization. (2022). *History of hospice.* https://www.nhpco.org/hospice-care-overview/history-of-hospice/

National Institute on Aging. (2021). *Providing care and comfort at the end of life.* https://www.nia.nih.gov/health/providing-comfort-end-life

Norris, A. (1999). A pilot study of an outcome measure in palliative care. *International Journal of Palliative Nursing, 5,* 40–45. https://doi.org/10.12968/ijpn.1999.5.1.9931

Panchmatia, N., & Urch, C. (2014). The feasibility of using goal attainment scaling in an acute oncology setting. *European Journal of Palliative Care, 21,* 138–143.

Patient Protection and Affordable Care Act, Pub. L. 111-148, 42 U.S.C. §§ 18001–18121 (2010). https://www.congress.gov/111/plaws/publ148/PLAW-111publ148.pdf

Peoples, H., Brandt, A., Wæhrens, E. E., & la Cour, K. (2017). Managing occupations in everyday life for people with advanced cancer living at home. *Scandinavian Journal of Occupational Therapy, 24,* 57–64. https://doi.org/10.1080/11038128.2016.1225815

Pickens, N. D. (2011). Grief and bereavement. In G. Stoffel & C. Brown (Eds.), *Occupational therapy in mental health: A vision for participation* (pp. 764–772). F. A. Davis.

Pizzi, M. A., & Richards, L. G. (2017). Promoting health, well-being, and quality of life in occupational therapy: A commitment to a paradigm shift for the next 100 years. *American Journal of Occupational Therapy, 71,* 7104170010. https://doi.org/10.5014/ajot.2017.028456

Reisberg, B. (1984). Functional Assessment Staging Tool (FAST). *Psychopharmacology Bulletin, 4,* 653–659.

Rickerson, E., Harrold, J., Kapo, J., Carroll, J. T., & Casarett, D. (2005). Timing of hospice referral and families' perceptions of services: Are earlier hospice referrals better? *Journal of the American Geriatrics Society, 53,* 819–823. https://doi.org/10.1111/j.1532-5415.2005.53259.x

Sakaguchi, S., & Okamura, H. (2015). Effectiveness of collage activity based on a life review in elderly cancer patients: A preliminary study. *Palliative and Supportive Care, 13,* 285–293. https://doi.org/10.1017/S1478951514000194

Schockett, E. R., Teno, J. M., Miller, S. C., & Stuart, B. (2005). Late referral to hospice and bereaved family member perception of quality of end-of-life care. *Journal of Pain and Symptom Management, 30,* 400–407. https://doi.org/10.1016/j.jpainsymman.2005.04.013

Siebert, C. (2022). *The hidden context of practice with older adults: Medicare policy, payment & monitoring* [Lecture PowerPoint slides]. Contact carol@the-home-remedy.com for access.

Singer, P. A., Martin, D. K., & Kelner, M. (1999). Quality end-of-life care: Patients' perspectives. *JAMA, 281*(2), 163–168. https://doi.org/10.1001/jama.281.2.163

Steinhauser, K. E., Christakis, N. A., Clipp, E. C., McNeilly, M., McIntyre, L., & Tulsky, J. A. (2000). Factors considered important at the end of life by patients, family, physicians, and other care providers. *JAMA, 284,* 2476–2482. https://www.doi.org/10.1001/jama.284.19.2476

Sviden, G. A., Tham, K., & Borell, L. (2010). Involvement in everyday life for people with a life-threatening illness. *Palliative and Supportive Care, 8,* 345–352. https://doi.org/10.1017/S1478951510000143

Szabat, M., & Knox, J. B. L. (2021). Shades of hope: Marcel's notion of hope in end-of-life care. *Medicine, Health Care, and Philosophy, 24,* 529–542. https://doi.org/10.1007/s11019-021-10036-1

Talbot-Coulombe, C., & Guay, M. (2020). Occupational therapy training on palliative and end-of-life care: Scoping review. *British Journal of Occupational Therapy, 83,* 609–619. https://doi.org/10.1177%2F0308022620926935

Taylor, D. H., Ostermann, J., Van Houtven, C. H., Tulsky, J. A., & Steinhauser, K. (2007). What length of hospice use maximizes reduction in medical expenditures near death in the US Medicare program? *Social Science and Medicine, 65,* 1466–1478. https://doi.org/10.1016/j.socscimed.2007.05.028

Teno, J. M., Shu, J. E., Casarett, D., Spence, C., Rhodes, R., & Connor, S. (2007). Timing of referral to hospice and quality of care: Length of stay and bereaved family members' perceptions of the timing of hospice referral. *Journal of Pain and Symptom Management, 34,* 120–125. https://doi.org/10.1016/j.jpainsymman.2007.04.014

Vossel, H. (2021). Getting upstream: A hospice playbook for value-based care. *Hospice News.* https://www.communityhospice.com/about/media-room/getting-upstream-a-hospice-playbook-for-value-based-care/

Yamaga, T., Asano, K., Ikeya, M., & Nakanishi, K. (2021). Successful occupational therapy at end of life for a patient with prostate sarcoma. *BMJ Case Reports, 14,* e242056. https://doi.org/10.1136/bcr-2021-242056

Yeh, H. E., & McColl, M. A. (2019). A model for occupation-based palliative care. *Occupational Therapy in Health Care, 33,* 108–123. https://doi.org/10.1080/07380577.2018.1544428

Yerxa, E. (1998). Health and the human spirit for occupation. *American Journal of Occupational Therapy, 52,* 412–418. https://doi.org/10.5014/ajot.52.6.412

5

Delivering Occupational Therapy Services in Palliative Care

LINDSEY BUDDELMEYER, OTD, MOT, OTR/L, and ANDREA SENSEL, OTD, OTR/L

Learning Objectives

After completing this chapter, readers will be able to

- explain the relevance and paradigm of occupational therapy and valued occupations in palliative care;
- discuss how occupational therapy practitioners are treating the chronic disease community in already-established pathways;
- recognize the culture and application of palliative care practice;
- describe the role of occupational therapy in palliative care;
- share examples of models of practice, assessments, goals, plan of care, and interventions commonly used by occupational therapists in palliative care;
- state the billing practices for palliative care; and
- explain a case example to demonstrate the application of occupational therapy services for a patient and caregiver receiving palliative care.

Key Terms and Concepts

adaptive equipment
Area Agencies on Aging
CAPABLE
caregiver education
diagnosis-specific organizations
energy conservation strategies

faith-based supports
Functional Assessment Staging Tool
Habitat for Humanity
HARP
health management
home modifications
occupational therapy evaluation
occupational therapy interventions
palliative care
Person–Environment–Occupation model
Skills2Care™
Zarit Burden Interview

The words *palliative care* and *hospice* are often used interchangeably by both health care professionals and the lay community, and there is evidence to support the perception that Americans believe that palliative care and hospice are equivalent (Ornstein et al., 2016). However, they are two separate delivery models with distinct differences that must be recognized to best serve those facing chronic illness and end-of-life care. In addition, there is misinformation regarding when and for whom palliative care services are most beneficial. These factors all contribute to whether palliative care, hospice care, or both are recommended and to whether patients, caregivers, and families are open to receiving them.

This chapter further delineates what separates palliative care from hospice and shares information about the *Occupational Therapy Practice Framework: Domain and Process* (4th ed.; *OTPF–4;* American Occupational Therapy Association [AOTA], 2020) with the case examples of Sandy. This information should provide readers with a deeper level of understanding in relation to ongoing care and what is oftentimes referred to as a *continuum of care.* The details involved in this type of care such as eligibility, referral, implementation of care, and discharge or referral to hospice care when appropriate will be provided. After reading this chapter, readers will be able to more clearly understand and recognize the distinct value that occupational therapy brings to the palliative care team.

Case Example 5.1 introduces the case of Sandy. This case demonstrates both the strength and the beauty of what can transpire when patients and families are supported from the beginning to the end of their journey with chronic illness.

Referral to Palliative Care: Eligibility and Initiation of Care

According to *Families Caring for an Aging America* (National Academies of Sciences, Engineering, and Medicine, 2016), there are millions of

CASE EXAMPLE 5.1. SANDY: INTRODUCTION

"We don't know what to do. Our mother is undoubtedly showing signs of Alzheimer's disease, and our dad is suffering too. We do not know how to help both of them. Can occupational therapy help us?"

Meet **Sandy,** a 70-year-old Caucasian woman; her husband John; and their two daughters, Jodi and Julie. At the time of this discussion, Sandy's husband and two daughters were at a point of uncertainty, fear, and confusion. Sandy was struggling with her memory, John was struggling to understand, and their two daughters were trying their best to make sense of everything and, most important, how to help both of them. No formal diagnosis had yet been given, which many times is critical to unlocking some level of support and care.

After an initial occupational therapy consult with the family, Sandy was soon diagnosed with the beginning stages of Alzheimer's disease (AD) by her primary care physician. Although this was not the diagnosis they wanted to hear, now they knew for certain what they were dealing with. It was time to figure out a way to best support this patient and her family.

Americans who provide some level of care and support to an older neighbor, friend, spouse, or older parent due to a limitation in their cognitive, mental, or physical abilities. With chronic disease, myriad physical, mental, and social challenges negatively affect patients, caregivers, family members, and friends (Harris & Wallace, 2012). ***Palliative care*** is a model of care that involves serving all people affected by and caring for someone facing chronic illness. According to the World Health Organization (2022), palliative care is focused on relieving suffering and improving quality of life (QoL) for all persons facing chronic illness. Palliative care has demonstrated its added value to the medical community as research has shown it to be more effective in comparison to standard approaches (Gunten, 2012). In addition, studies involving a true interdisciplinary palliative care intervention demonstrate improved QoL for patients as well as cost savings (Milazzo et al., 2020). Although the literature is strong with respect to palliative care practice with the oncology community, anyone diagnosed with a chronic illness is eligible to receive palliative care services (Bhatnagar & Patel, 2018).

According to the Center to Advance Palliative Care (2020), five pillars provide structure to the work in palliative care:

- expert symptom management to reduce both physical and emotional distress
- consultation support for primary care providers and specialists in caring for their most complex patients
- skilled communication and intensive patient, family, and clinician decision-making discussions
- clear patient and caregiver education on what to expect to empower patients to handle symptoms at home, enable optimal shared decision making, and reduce anxiety
- coordinated care and efficient transitions across settings so that treatments match the changing needs and priorities of the patient and the family over the long course of a disease. (p. 7)

The process to initiate and receive palliative care is similar to the process required to receive traditional skilled care. Patients must be diagnosed with a chronic condition, and a physician must complete an order or prescription requesting occupational therapy and palliative care services (see Case Example 5.2). Patients and families have the ability to choose whatever palliative care organization they prefer. Once the referral is processed by the organization's intake staff, palliative care services are initiated. The first visit may include the physician, provider, and therapist. The order of service may be determined by the organization and any guidelines set forth by third-party payers. Patients who are eligible to receive palliative care services are able to stay under this model of care for as long as is medically necessary. The process of discharging because a patient has reached their maximum rehabilitative potential is simply not a part of this culture. The functional status of people living with chronic illness is expected to fluctuate. Palliative care services are able to align with the patient's needs on the basis of their stage of illness.

Addressing Meaningful Occupations Through Interventions

A core belief of the occupational therapy profession is that all people have an innate desire to engage in daily occupations. Occupations are viewed in relation to all of the daily tasks that occupy people's time. According to the *OTPF–4* (AOTA, 2020), occupational therapy practitioners may provide interventions for persons, groups, and populations in nine identified areas of occupation: ADLs, IADLs, health management, rest and sleep,

CASE EXAMPLE 5.2. SANDY: ALZHEIMER'S DISEASE DIAGNOSIS

After receiving a diagnosis of AD, Sandy was clearly a candidate for palliative care services. As are many Americans, she and her family were unaware of palliative care and what this model of care involved. Once they were educated on how palliative care would provide wraparound services to help manage her symptoms, provide education and support to the family, and include an interdisciplinary team of providers with a focus on improving QoL, they were all onboard—everyone, that is, except the patient. However, Sandy was open to allowing the occupational therapist to come in for an evaluation to meet with her and to discuss things further. This would prove to be a defining moment between her and the therapist. In reality, Sandy was not at a stage of acceptance in which she could have an open and honest dialogue about her memory and the fact that she had been diagnosed with AD. The therapist was respectful of this and was very intentional in meeting Sandy at her stage of acceptance of her illness. The therapist provided basic information about how palliative care services could best support both her and her family. The ultimate goal was to keep her home and be surrounded by her family whom she adored. Ultimately, the therapist and Sandy developed a strong therapeutic relationship, and she even began to look forward to the time they would spend together during their palliative care visits.

education, work, play, leisure, and social participation. Each of these occupations holds different value and meaning for every person, including those with chronic conditions.

Studies have shown that people who stop engaging in daily activities experience poor mental and physical health and decreased overall QoL (Mackichan et al., 2013). Occupational therapy practitioners add value to the palliative care team by supporting people in their ability to lead fulfilling lives within the constraints of their illness (Eva & Morgan, 2018). This important work is done by addressing and attacking barriers that impede patients and their ability to engage in valued life roles and daily occupations (AOTA, 2015b). Depending on the stage of the chronic illness, practitioners may focus their goals in the following areas (note that this is not an exhaustive list) in relation to meaningful occupations:

- addressing challenges in ADLs and home management tasks to help enhance the ability to improve participation and level of independence in these areas

- providing strategies, including energy conservation techniques and grading or adapting activities, to make up for the physical demands and decrease the fatigue associated with many chronic conditions
- individualizing adaptations for patients to perform health management tasks (i.e., daily insulin shots for diabetes)
- teaching and incorporating ***health management*** tasks into current habits and patterns of behaviors so that they become a part of the daily routine (e.g., a medication reminder system)
- addressing physical and psychosocial health and well-being by helping patients develop effective coping strategies, habits, routines, behaviors, and adaptations to their lifestyle. (AOTA, 2015a, p. 1)

Occupational therapy practitioners are trained to be occupation focused and may use occupations as both a means and an end to achieve therapeutic gains. On completion of an evaluation and analysis, practitioners choose an approach to further guide the intervention process. These approaches include creating and promoting, establishing and restoring, maintaining, modifying, and preventing disability. The approach allows practitioners to use a model or models of practice that will be most useful to guide the pathway for patients and caregivers to do the things that they need and want to do in a day's time.

Most, if not all, chronic disease communities experience some level of challenge in the participation and completion of daily occupations. This is when the purpose of the occupational therapy profession becomes ever clearer, and the occupational therapy practitioner becomes even more important to have on the care team. Practitioners assess what is and is not working for patients and caregivers in terms of daily routines. They do this collaboratively with patients and caregivers to determine where to start bridging this gap. There is a deliberate and intentional effort to allow patients and families to feel heard and to figure out a way to empower and support them (see Case Example 5.3). A core and fundamental wish that practitioners have for their patients and families is that they will be able to live a purposeful and meaningful life, no matter what illness or difficult circumstances they may be facing.

Common Care Challenges for the Patient and Caregiver

Occupations that implicitly involve two or more people may be termed *co-occupations* (Zemke & Clark, 1996). According to the *OTPF–4,* caregiving

CASE EXAMPLE 5.3. SANDY: IADL OF DRIVING

When the occupational therapist was initially working with Sandy, she was experiencing a great deal of anxiety and frustration with changes she had noticed in her memory. She was tight lipped about her diagnosis and asked that her family be respectful of where she was at in her ability to openly discuss it. The therapist continued to honor where Sandy was at in her journey with AD but made an effort to slowly and methodically educate both her and her family on facts versus myths about her illness. This important work was done in tandem through the integration of valued occupations.

The first task at hand was to address an incredibly meaningful IADL, driving. At the time of the evaluation, Sandy was still performing this occupation independently. However, her family shared that they were very concerned that she was unsafe to drive. She had gotten lost several times, and her thinking appeared to be increasingly scattered. The occupational therapist agreed to assess this area further and also recommended that she complete a driving evaluation. The therapist pulled in a resource from the The Hartford (2022), "At the Crossroads: Family Conversations About Alzheimer's Disease, Dementia, and Driving." She sat down with Sandy and asked her to complete the "Driving Behavior Warning Signs—When Noticed, How Often" worksheet. Through this exercise, it soon became clear that Sandy was not going to push back against her family for no longer wanting her to drive. Rather, she too had secretly become fearful of driving. Therefore, instead of telling Sandy she should not drive anymore, the therapist used a strategy to empower Sandy: She offered a safe space for her to come to this conclusion on her own.

At the same time, the occupational therapist explained to both Sandy and her family how compromised her executive functioning skills had become as a result of her illness. Attention was drawn to the fact that with AD, changes are typically gradual and can be difficult to detect and capture in real time. Driving required more abilities than Sandy had at this point, which was by no means her fault. In the end, a formal driving evaluation was no longer necessary. The patient and family had a better understanding of the physiological changes in the brain associated with AD. Everyone rallied around Sandy and agreed to take her wherever she needed to go. She focused on the fact that she would be able to spend even more time with her family, which was very important and meaningful to her.

is considered a co-occupation. This involves active participation by both the caregiver and the care recipient (AOTA, 2020). It is important to recognize that although caregiving may be a valued co-occupation for some, it may be an act of obligation or duty for others. This can certainly affect the dynamics involved with care.

Most caregivers have no formal education or training to understand how to care for their loved one with chronic illness. In fact, people with chronic illness and their respective caregivers may lack ongoing and sustainable skilled support and services. Often, they do not qualify for skilled services involving what are most commonly known to other professionals and the community as *rehabilitation specialists* (i.e., occupational therapy, physical therapy, speech therapy). The patient's level of function at the onset of illness cannot be restored, so people assume that there is no therapeutic gain to involving a therapy team. However, occupational therapy can add value and support for the patient and family to address barriers and challenges that affect their everyday life activities in step with the chronic and progressive nature of their illness.

An important belief in palliative care is that the needs of both the patient and the caregiver must be addressed. There is recognition that meeting the patient's daily needs depends on the caregiver. Palliative care practice is designed to be both patient and caregiver driven. To treat one and not the other would be a disservice to both and would not reflect best practice in working with the chronic disease community. In fact, family caregivers of older adults with chronic disease are tasked with many hardships and health risks related to this occupational role, which in turn influences their overall QoL, health, and well-being (Mthembu et al., 2016).

Patients and caregivers face a wide range of daily functional challenges depending on the stage and state of the patient's illness (see Case Example 5.4). However, occupational therapy practitioners may need to address more common care challenges among patients and caregivers that are worth noting. The information in Table 5.1 may be used by all health care disciplines to better understand some examples of when an occupational therapy palliative care referral may be appropriate and warranted.

Evaluation

The ***occupational therapy evaluation*** process in palliative care is similar to traditional practice. The evaluation template has a placeholder for standard types of information such as primary diagnosis, secondary conditions, occupational profile information, and musculoskeletal and

CASE EXAMPLE 5.4. SANDY'S CAREGIVER

Health management was an important area of occupation for Sandy that required immediate attention. There was an increasing need to address medication management. Daily completion of this task was overwhelming and becoming unmanageable for both John and Sandy. The occupational therapist assessed current practice and routine for the patient and caregiver and determined that John believed that Sandy was taking her medication when he set it out for her when in actuality she was not. He did not want to control or take another thing away from her, but she was simply having difficulty remembering to take her pills despite his efforts to set them out as a visual reminder to her.

The occupational therapist continued to educate John on the fact that Sandy's memory challenges were such that he needed to take more of a leadership role in the daily management of her care. This can be a difficult concept for caregivers because they most easily identify with the role that the patient has previously played—in this case, for the past 50 years. Sandy had been completely independent in every area of occupation until AD. However, through collaboration and further understanding of the disease, John began to embrace this role. The therapist, patient, and caregiver created a daily routine that would meet both John's and Sandy's needs to order, dispense, and manage all of Sandy's medications. A 7-day medication management pill dispenser was issued, and John was shown how to use his phone alarm to set reminders to give Sandy her medications at the appropriate times. Again, the therapist, patient, and caregiver collaborated to identify strategies that would support their active lifestyle while improving the safety and management of Sandy's medications.

ADLs specifically involving bathing, dressing, and grooming were areas that had become increasingly difficult for both Sandy and John to manage. Sandy was losing her ability to self-initiate and complete daily tasks independently, and John was growing more discouraged as he watched his wife struggle with what were once simple daily tasks. Sandy had a beauty routine that she engaged in daily that was meaningful and important to her. This routine involved styling her hair, applying makeup, and picking out her clothes on the basis of the season and day's events. She was a beautiful woman and exuded a classic sense of style. This was simply a part of who she was and who her family knew and loved. Unfortunately, through time, her ADL routine became a more burdensome task, and she was limited in her ability to begin and complete these tasks independently.

Sandy eventually lost the ability to pick out an outfit and to dress and undress independently. The occupational therapist and John worked together to reshape

(Continued)

CASE EXAMPLE 5.4. SANDY'S CAREGIVER *(Cont.)*

the way he approached this ADL with his wife so that he again took more of the lead to help support her participation in what was once a valued occupation. With the help and support of his daughters, specific outfits were organized on hangers for Sandy on the basis of the current season. All other nonseasonal clothes were placed in a separate closet to avoid confusing and overwhelming Sandy. In terms of dressing, the therapist recommended and worked with John and their two daughters to put together a dressing and sequencing book for Sandy. John was educated to put this out in front of his wife once he had gathered her clothes and to refer her to this book to give her an additional visual cue to complete the task. At the time, John shared that he did not feel like this would do much in terms of helping her, but that he would at least try it. To his surprise, this adaptation was a success. Sandy was able to follow along with the dressing and sequencing book and participated successfully and willingly in dressing. This not only made Sandy feel empowered to engage more, but it also made John feel a sense of joy and pride to see that his wife was still quite capable when she was provided the appropriate level of support, modifications, and adaptations.

TABLE 5.1. Specific Care Challenges: How Occupational Therapy Can Help

Care Challenge or Area of Occupation	Meaning of Identified Area	Examples of What OTPs Could Specifically Address
Difficulty in the ability to engage in daily functional tasks	Performing everyday life activities that the patient needs and wants to do	Bed mobility, dressing, bathing, and toileting
Difficulty with or decreased functional and community mobility	Navigating safely and independently through the home and the community	Fall prevention strategies, driving assessments, environmental and safety assessments, positioning, and recommending mobility devices to increase comfort and safety
Difficulty with meal preparation and home management	Difficulty preparing a snack or meal, handling daily operations of the home	Doing laundry, house cleaning, care of pets

(Continued)

TABLE 5.1. Specific Care Challenges: How Occupational Therapy Can Help *(Cont.)*

Care Challenge or Area of Occupation	Meaning of Identified Area	Examples of What OTPs Could Specifically Address
Difficulty with health management	Challenges with symptom management, such as fatigue, pain, anxiety, or shortness of breath; attending regularly scheduled doctor's appointments; handling medication management and refills	Medication management, fatigue-related issues, pain, anxiety
Difficulty with rest and sleep patterns	Difficulty with preparing for bedtime, safety concerns with sleep routine, poor sleep patterns	Establishment of habit and routine for sleep preparation, environmental assessment for safety when sleeping and getting up to toilet during the night, safe practice for sleep participation, incontinence supplies
Difficulty or lack of interest in leisure	Decreased or lack of interest in engaging in or doing things that were once pleasurable hobbies or leisure interests	Adaptation to leisure interests, exploration of different leisure pursuits, education and training with caregiver to assist with leisure exploration and participation

Note. OTPs = occupational therapy practitioners.

cognitive functioning. An important difference to note in the occupational therapy palliative care evaluation is in the plan-of-care and goals sections. The focus is more habilitative; therefore, goals are made for much longer periods of time. This better reflects a maintenance type of approach and need for ongoing support and servicing. Similar to traditional practice, goals may be patient focused, caregiver focused, or both.

Specific assessments or screens appropriate to use during the evaluation may be determined by the occupational therapist and palliative care team. More commonly used assessments may be embedded into the evaluation template for increased ease and use. For example, dementia is a common condition in the chronic disease community. Therefore, the Montreal Cognitive Assessment (Nasreddine et al., 2005) may be an agreed-on baseline standard of measure of cognitive functioning that the palliative care team uses in the beginning stages of evaluation and assessment with a patient. In addition, there are also assessments that are more commonly understood across disciplines that may be used to further assess the stage of the patient's illness and to offer an objective measure of when it may be time to transition to hospice care.

FUNCTIONAL ASSESSMENT STAGING SCALE

In keeping with the case example, AD, which is the most common form of dementia, has a very predictable pattern of progression that is laid out in an assessment called the ***Functional Assessment Staging Tool*** (FAST) scale. The FAST is an observational scale that describes a continuum of seven successive stages of dementia, from normal to the most severe stage (Reisberg, 1988). According to Sclan and Reisberg (1992), the FAST is a reliable and valid assessment technique for evaluating functional deterioration in patients with AD from the beginning to the end of their illness. Moreover, the results suggest that the FAST provides a characteristic pattern of functional decline associated with AD.

ZARIT BURDEN INTERVIEW

A comprehensive evaluation of patients with chronic disease should also include the caregiver. A commonly used assessment tool to evaluate caregiver burden in order to provide supportive services and resources is the ***Zarit Burden Interview.*** The original interview was developed in 1980 and consists of 29 statements; caregivers rated their agreement with each statement on a scale ranging from 0 (*never*) to 4 (*almost always*). Since 1980, multiple versions of the tool have been published, including 12-item and 6-item shorter scales to decrease administration time. A study by Yu et al. (2018) found that the 6-item and 12-item versions demonstrated diagnostic outcomes similar to those of the original 29-item version and can be easily and quickly administered to caregivers during evaluation. Examples of statements caregivers are asked to rate on a scale of 0 (*never*) to 4 (*almost always*), in all versions of the assessment include, "You don't have enough time for yourself," "You are stressed between caregiving and meeting other responsibilities," and "Caregiving affects your relationship with others in a negative way." The ratings for all statements in the assessment are added, and scores are placed into categories ranging from *no burden* to *severe burden*. The Zarit Burden Interview is a quick and easy method to gain important evaluation data to plan interventions to support patients and their caregivers in thriving at home.

Intervention

Care plans for ***occupational therapy interventions*** in palliative care are as unique and diverse as the patients served. Occupational therapy practitioners strive to provide interventions to support QoL and independence in functional tasks that are meaningful to the patient. Many times, to support patients' goals, interventions also need to incorporate family, friends, and caregivers. Common and critical elements of many palliative care occupational therapy interventions include home modifications, assistive technology, energy conservation, and caregiver education.

Creating an environment supportive of a patient's current and future occupational performance is a foundational aspect of palliative care intervention. Occupational therapy practitioners' extensive knowledge of chronic disease management and progression and their impacts on occupational performance allows for interventions that include home environment evaluations and modifications. Forward planning and modifications can help provide a home environment that will support a patient and caregiver throughout the progression of the disease.

HOME MODIFICATIONS

Home modifications are defined as individually tailored interventions that eliminate barriers and promote the client's independence in everyday tasks (Granbom et al., 2017). Interventions for occupational engagement are highly individualized on the basis of the client's personal factors identified during evaluation. Personal factor considerations during the home modification process, as discussed by Stark et al. (2011), include the client's health condition, readiness for change, terms of housing occupancy, financial resources, and type of solution. When providing care to people with chronic disease, it is important not only to consider their current functional status but also to plan for future abilities and difficulties.

For example, when making recommendations for home modifications to increase independence with functional mobility with a walker for a patient with Parkinson's disease, it is important not only to plan for walker clearance and access throughout vital parts of the home but also to consider the progressive nature of the disease and make recommendations that will accommodate a wheelchair. A client's readiness for change is also an important piece of information to consider while making home modification recommendations.

If a client and their family are still in the precontemplative stage of change and not ready to accept the need for change, home modification recommendations may not be well received and can affect the client–therapist relationship. Additional things to consider before making home modification recommendations include whether the patient is renting or owns their home, the financial resources the client has available to make changes, and the type and invasiveness of the modifications recommended.

Home modifications can range in involvement, with classifications ranging from simple to complex. Simple home modifications are defined as nonstructural or simple structural modifications or do-it-yourself projects that are low in complexity (Ainsworth & de Jonge, 2019). They can also include home repairs and maintenance that support home safety and independence. In contrast, a complex modification involves major structural changes to a home that typically require a professional for completion. Again, in offering solutions to support occupational engagement, it is imperative to consider a client's readiness for change, financial resources, and health condition. The following are lists of simple and complex home modifications frequently used to help maximize patient independence.

Simple home modifications

- installing grab bars next to the toilet to increase ease of clothing management and transfers
- adding a handrail at the main entrance to the house to increase independence with access to the mailbox
- changing from door knobs to levers to decrease pain when opening or closing a bedroom door
- installing slip-resistant flooring or slip-resistant strips in the bathroom to decrease fall risk while bathing

- adding shelving to the living room to remove clutter from the floor and placing commonly used items in easy-to-reach areas to decrease the risk of falls
- lowering closet rods or shelving to increase ease of access from wheelchair level during dressing tasks
- moving items commonly used in the kitchen from higher shelves to lower shelves or countertop storage.

Complex home modifications

- adding a permanent ramp to the front of the home for wheelchair access to and from the home
- widening doorways to allow for walker and wheelchair clearance into bathrooms and bedrooms
- remodeling the kitchen to provide countertop and appliance access from a seated position
- updating the bathroom from a tub shower to a walk-in shower
- replacing standard-height toilets with comfort-height toilets to increase ease of sit-to-stand transfers.

ADAPTIVE EQUIPMENT

Recommending and educating patients receiving palliative care and patients with chronic disease on the use of adaptive equipment to increase the ease of daily occupations that are important to them is another common intervention used by occupational therapy practitioners. ***Adaptive equipment*** is defined as devices used to compensate for a physical limitation to promote safety and prevent injury while completing ADLs (Koketsu, 2018). Adaptive equipment can be purchased off the shelf or online, or items the patient already owns can be adapted with a little creativity. Online resources such as Pinterest and AOTA discussion boards can spark the occupational therapy practitioner's imagination to create low-cost, personalized solutions for clients. Listed here are just a few adaptive equipment ideas to help promote occupational engagement.

Functional mobility

- adding a basket or tray to a walker to assist with item retrieval and mobility

- building up walker or cane handles with foam to increase ease of grip
- adding colored tape to wheelchair brakes for easy location.

Bathing, dressing, and grooming

- reacher, sock aid, elastic shoelaces, and shoehorn education to decrease the need to bend over for dressing tasks
- tub transfer bench, handheld shower, grab bars, and soap in pantyhose tied to the grab bar to increase independence in bathing and prevent losing the soap
- built-up grooming utensils, electric toothbrush, and mounted fingernail clippers and nail file for nail care.

Toileting

- elevated toilet seat or bedside commode
- wiping aids such as tongs, wet wipes, or Bottom Buddy
- loops on pants to help with lower body clothing management after toileting.

Meal preparation and eating

- built-up utensils using foam curlers or tubes
- plates and bowls with side guards
- utility cart to assist with item retrieval and mobility.

Leisure

- card holder for managing and manipulating playing cards
- extra-large or color-coded television remote
- long-handled items for pet care, such as food and water bowl or a cat litter box scoop.

ENERGY CONSERVATION STRATEGIES

In addition to promoting continued engagement in daily tasks through home modifications and adaptive equipment, education on and implementing energy conservation strategies into a patient's daily routine can be very beneficial. ***Energy conservation strategies*** are any modification to a task that reduces the energy expenditure required for its completion (Wingardh, 2020). Assisting patients with implementing energy conservation strategies into their daily routine can help them to continue to maintain occupational independence as well as to engage in leisure occupations.

A study conducted by Wingardh et al. (2020) to examine the effectiveness of energy conservation education with patients with chronic obstructive pulmonary disease (COPD) found that a 2-week education program on energy conservation techniques reduced patients' energy expenditure while completing ADL tasks without any significant change in the time spent on task completion. This finding is similar to an earlier study completed by Mathiowetz et al. (2005), who examined the effectiveness of energy conservation education with patients diagnosed with multiple sclerosis. As in the study conducted with patients with COPD, patients with multiple sclerosis demonstrated substantial benefits from implementing energy conservation strategies into their daily routine, with results indicating a reduction in scores on both the Physical and Social subscales of the Fatigue Impact Scale (Mathiowetz et al., 2005). Common energy conservation strategies occupational therapy practitioners can assist patients to incorporate into their daily routines include but are certainly not limited to

- completing ADL tasks seated instead of standing to decrease energy expenditure,
- using proper body mechanics,
- scheduling tasks to be completed strategically throughout the day with rest breaks to avoid exhaustion,
- planning ahead (e.g., getting clothing items for dressing out the night before, making larger batches of meals to eat throughout the week, scheduling appointments or trips to the store during less busy days),
- moving commonly used items to low cabinets or countertops for easy access,
- bathing with warm water instead of hot water to avoid shortness of breath,
- using long-handled items for ADLs (e.g., reachers, long-handled shoe horns, dust pans) to decrease bending, and
- breathing strategies to help combat shortness of breath.

CAREGIVER EDUCATION

A final but significant intervention method used during occupational therapy treatment is ***caregiver education.*** For many patients with chronic disease, an informal caregiver is an important member of their health care team. Informal caregivers may aid in tasks ranging from running errands, household management, and meal preparation to assistance with basic ADLs. Educating and empowering caregivers with the strategies and knowledge to best support their loved ones will not only lead to increased ease in day-to-day routines but also to improved outcomes for the patient. In a study examining the effectiveness of family-based education on outcomes for persons with Type 2 diabetes, a significant reduction was found in A1C levels and body mass index, as well as a significant increase in patient self-efficacy, when extensive education was provided to the family unit (Cai & Hu, 2016). Strategies to incorporate caregiver education into intervention sessions include scheduling appointment times when caregivers can attend, encouraging active caregiver participation in treatment, keeping a log of recommendations and resources for easy caregiver access, and actively seeking feedback from caregivers regarding areas of concern and progress.

Using Models of Practice and Evidence To Guide Thinking

Ecological models, such as the Person–Environment–Occupation (PEO) model, are helpful tools that can be used to help guide practitioners in decision making to help maximize patients' safety and independence in the home. The ***PEO model*** considers three factors—the person, the environment, and the occupation—and how the interaction among these factors influences occupational performance (Strong & Rebeiro, 2011). Assessing strengths and barriers in each of these areas and providing intervention strategies that address the barriers can help to promote occupational performance.

For example, a client diagnosed with congestive heart failure was referred for an occupational therapy evaluation because of difficulty with bathing. Using the PEO model for guidance, the occupational therapist evaluated the patient's strength, cognition, and home environment and the context in which the patient was completing her bathing. Barriers were identified as decreased strength, a tub shower with no handrails or seat, and attempting to complete the ADL standing. The interaction of these barriers was affecting the patient's ability to perform the occupation of bathing. A treatment plan was developed and implemented to address these barriers and to help promote independence with bathing tasks.

Home modification—a direct focus on the environment and how patients interact within it—is a common intervention strategy used by occupational therapy practitioners to promote patient independence in daily activities and safety in the home. Although many of these interventions occur organically throughout care sessions, the literature discusses two standardized home modification programs, CAPABLE (Community Aging in Place—Advancing Better Living for Elders) and HARP (Home Hazard Removal Program), that have demonstrated effectiveness in randomized trials.

CAPABLE

CAPABLE is a 10-session, home-based interprofessional program that includes an occupational therapist, a nurse, and a handyman. This team helps to address older adults' self-identified goals by enhancing individual capabilities and the home environment (Szanton et al., 2021). In a randomized trial with 1,144 community-dwelling older adults with disabilities and 4,236 matched comparators, those who participated in the CAPABLE program demonstrated improvements in ADLs and IADLs with strong to large effect sizes (Szanton et al., 2021).

HARP

Similarly, ***HARP*** is a fall prevention intervention implemented by an occupational therapist that includes a comprehensive assessment, home modification recommendations, assistance with removing home hazards, and fall prevention education. In a randomized clinical trial published in 2021, participants who participated in HARP demonstrated a reduced rate of falls compared with the control group (Stark et al., 2021). Both of these programs demonstrate the value and importance of occupational therapy in addressing barriers in the home environment to support and maximize occupational performance.

SKILLS2CARE

Skills2Care™ is a program that was developed and researched by Dr. Laura Gitlin and her research team at Thomas Jefferson University. The focus of this program is to provide home-based occupational therapy services for caregivers who are providing informal caregiving services for a loved one with dementia. Skills2Care is a collaborative model that is driven by the caregiver for the caregiver, with the formalized guidance and support of an occupational therapy practitioner.

Skills2Care is theory driven (stress process theories and competence–environmental press and environmental vulnerability frameworks) and has been tested using randomized trial methodology (Jefferson Elder Care, 2022). It is a nonpharmacological intervention that is focused on recognizing and responding to environmental triggers and behavioral manifestations that commonly occur among the population with dementia. This program may be used solely with the caregiver or in conjunction with the caregiver and care recipient. The Skills2Care program approaches the chronic nature of dementia by educating caregivers about the disease process, identifying and implementing strategies to identify and respond to behavioral challenges, making necessary occupational shifts as clients with AD become more disconnected from past leisure pursuits and interests, taking care of the self to manage caregiver stressors, and feeling more confident in caregiving responsibilities, communication skills, and activity simplification strategies that all feed into the overall well-being and health of clients with dementia and their caregivers. Although the Skills2Care program has traditionally been delivered under a home health model of care, it is important to note that these services may also be embedded under a palliative care model, which would afford patients and caregivers the ability to receive specialized care and training in an ongoing way to better align with the chronic and progressive nature of the illness.

The Skills2Care program has been successfully implemented in both a home health and palliative care model design. Occupational therapy practitioners might consider the services they provide in more traditional models of practice and ask themselves: Is there a space for them in palliative care?

Resources to Support the Chronic Disease Community

Advocating for access to services and resources are critical components of supporting patients with chronic disease. For patients to continue to engage in daily occupations, it is important for occupational therapy practitioners to be aware of and be able to educate patients and their families on local, state, and national resources available. Resources may be available from both traditional medically based organizations and community-based organizations.

MEDICALLY BASED RESOURCES

Medically based resources are typically better understood and more frequently used to help support patients with chronic disease. These resources are traditionally taught in practitioner curricula, and they are often associated with the organization that is providing care. The interprofessional health care team is a key medically based resource to help support positive outcomes for patients. It is important that occupational therapy practitioners be able to understand other disciplines' scope of practice and refer accordingly to help support the patient when needed. Not only does each member of the team come with their own unique perspective on and expertise in supporting the patient, but they also provide holistic and comprehensive care for symptom management and continued occupational engagement.

In addition to proper utilization of the health care team, other medically based resources such as durable medical equipment (DME) providers, who have access to a wide range of DME that can help support function, can help to support patients with chronic disease. These providers also have a solid understanding of medical billing and can assist in navigating equipment coverage and reimbursement when appropriate.

FAITH-BASED SUPPORTS

Faith-based supports are a community-based support that can offer multiple supports and services. Once again, services vary on the basis of the community in which the patient lives; however, local churches or faith-based groups often offer very helpful support for patients with chronic disease. Many faith-based organizations receive donations of DME such as walkers, wheelchairs, tub benches, and reachers when a member of their congregation passes away, allowing for a lending closet of items that can be used at little to no cost. Many organizations also offer additional support opportunities such as short-term meal delivery, companion services, transportation, and assistance with simple home repairs.

Although this section offers examples and a discussion of medically and community-based resources to support patients with chronic diseases, it is important to recognize that this list is not exhaustive. Each community in which occupational therapy practitioners practice has its own unique network of supports, and the exploration of these supports requires a creative and open mind to fully support the patient (see Case Example 5.5).

COMMUNITY-BASED RESOURCES

Although not tapped into or considered as often, community-based resources also provide many valuable services to support continued occupational engagement of patients with chronic diseases. It is important that occupational therapy practitioners have an in-depth understanding of the unique services and organizations available in the communities they serve. One community-based resource that offers a wide variety of services to support older adults in specific geographical areas are local ***Area Agencies on Aging.*** Although specific services vary from agency to agency, common core services may include transportation, meal delivery services, care coordination, education, and household maintenance.

Many Area Agencies on Aging also have a supply or "loaner" closet of DME families have donated that can be used by patients. These agencies are a great way to locate resources such as walkers, wheelchairs, bedside commodes, and tub benches at little or no cost to the patient. For example, although most insurance covers one assistive device for a patient, multiple devices are sometimes needed for daily functional mobility. A patient with COPD who has already used their benefit for a wheelchair for most functional mobility throughout their home may need a rolling walker to access certain areas of the home such as the bathroom. If the patient does not have the financial ability to purchase a rolling walker out of pocket, the local Area Agency on Aging could be a great resource to help provide the much-needed equipment for continued independence with ADLs.

CASE EXAMPLE 5.5. SANDY: COMMUNITY RESOURCES

50 North, a senior center, was a community resource that provided a range of supports and services for John and Sandy. These resources were used at various stages of Sandy's illness. The first used was the Adaptive Equipment Donation service. Sandy began to struggle more and more with navigating safely in the bathroom, and John had to provide more and more physical assistance with grooming and bathing tasks. The occupational therapist thought that it was necessary to adapt the bathroom space to make things safer and more accessible for both Sandy and John. Therefore, higher-cost items such as a tub bench and raised toilet seat were checked out from the Adaptive Equipment Donation Center. This service was free to all community members living within county lines. Adaptive equipment could be kept by community members for as long as they needed it. Smaller-scale items such as an antiskid mat, grab bars, and a hand-held shower were purchased out of pocket. Low-level renovations and adaptations, which involved installation of a new hand-held removable shower head, removal of their heavy sliding shower doors, and hanging a new shower curtain rod and shower curtain, were completed by the Chore Services Department at 50 North. The time, labor, and cost for these services was less than $50, making it substantially more cost-efficient than using a contractor.

John also stepped into the newer role of having to plan and prepare meals for himself and his wife. This became burdensome for him on top of everything else that he was managing as the primary caregiver for his wife. Therefore, John and the occupational therapist collaborated and discussed the option of using Meals on Wheels, another resource offered through 50 North. This service provided hot meals for both John and his wife two times per week to help offset the weekly burden of John cooking every night. He appreciated this option and having further support to assist him in this important area of occupation.

Last, John joined the Male Caregiver Support Group offered at 50 North by the Alzheimer's Association. This was a space in which he was able to feel understood and supported in his endeavors as a spouse caring for his wife. His daughters took turns caring for Sandy so that he could attend the monthly support group. John formed relationships with other caregivers and learned new strategies that others found helpful as they all navigated various daily care challenges.

Habitat for Humanity is an additional community-based resource that can provide much-needed resources and services to people with chronic disease. Habitat for Humanity is a global nonprofit organization that works through local offices in all 50 states to support community members in building or improving a place they call home (Habitat for Humanity, 2022). Home repair services are offered to those who qualify on the basis of need and income. Services that patients with chronic diseases could benefit from include but are not limited to the installation of home safety equipment such as grab bars and hand railings for increased safety with functional transfers or building a ramp to allow access to and from a home for a person who uses a wheelchair at a reduced cost.

DIAGNOSIS-SPECIFIC ORGANIZATIONS

Diagnosis-specific organizations also offer a tremendous amount of support, education, and resources to patients with chronic disease and their families to assist with continued engagement in meaningful occupations. Although most diagnosis-specific organizations are national or global agencies, many have local sites to provide specialized education and recommendations to support patients with chronic disease based on the specific community's unique strengths. It is important that practitioners understand not only what broad services are offered in the community but also how additional community-specific agencies can help to supplement the care of patients.

One example of a diagnosis-specific organization that offers support is the Alzheimer's Association, which offers multiple support and educational opportunities at both the national and local levels for people with dementia. Examples of programming include an early-stage support group for patients newly diagnosed with mild cognitive impairment, caregiver support groups to provide education and engagement to people caring for loved ones with dementia, a free online education center with courses covering multiple topics related to living with and caring for someone with dementia, and care consultation services that provide coaching and support to families (Alzheimer's Association, 2022).

Similar to the Alzheimer's Association, the Parkinson's Foundation also provides support groups and educational opportunities for people diagnosed with Parkinson's disease. In addition to support and educational opportunities, the Parkinson's Foundation also offers valuable resources to patients and caregivers regarding specialized wellness, exercise, and comprehensive care centers in a patient's local area (Parkinson's Foundation, 2022).

Billing

Compared with other models of care, palliative care services are not considered profitable. However, this model of care involves more financial gains when one considers the role it plays in acting as a feeder system to both home health and hospice. Palliative care services are most frequently billed under Medicare Part B; however, they may also be billed through Medicare Advantage Organizations, private insurance, and Medicaid (Javens, 2021). Billing systems are set up and established on the basis of the organization's eligibility, the provider's credentialing, and regulatory guidelines. These will vary on the basis of the palliative care organization and its eligibility to bill for and receive payment for services. Appropriate billing codes and modifiers must be used as set forth by the most current billing and coding operations and procedure.

Occupational therapy practitioners should also consider grant-funding opportunities to support future endeavors involving occupational therapy's role in palliative care. A pilot program involving occupational therapy may help allocate time and space to explore the intricacies and logistical set-up of billing and coding for payment for occupational therapy services. In 2015, a grant was awarded by the Hancock County Community Foundation to a partnership between Blanchard Valley Health System and the University of Findlay in Findlay, Ohio, to pilot a palliative care program involving occupational therapy services for patients and caregivers facing dementia. This program was successfully implemented and ultimately led to training an additional two occupational therapy practitioners to deliver specialized care for patients with dementia under a palliative care model.

Challenges and Opportunities for Occupational Therapy Services in Palliative Care

Although the connection between occupational therapy and palliative care goals is apparent, the role of occupational therapy practitioners in palliative care is still considered an emerging area of practice. Although many challenges continue to exist in increasing occupational therapy's presence in palliative care, the opportunities make the case for the continued push into this area of practice.

Challenges need to be recognized and addressed in order to increase occupational therapy's presence and role in palliative care. First, there is a lack of understanding among the lay and professional communities regarding the true purpose and function of palliative care. This is a notable barrier with regard to others understanding occupational therapy's role. In addition, there is a lack of knowledge and understanding of palliative care eligibility, goals of care, and scope of practice. This limits the number of patients receiving palliative care services, as well as the wide range of interdisciplinary team members who could be used in this service line. Next, the stigma associated with receiving palliative care services is a barrier that needs to be confronted and broken down. A final challenge worth noting is the lack of traditional payment plans that cover skilled services under a maintenance model of care. Although some traditional coverage is available, exploring alternative funding sources such as grants should be sought out to continue to push the typical boundaries of where occupational therapy services have traditionally resided.

Although there continue to be challenges in providing occupational therapy services in palliative care, the opportunities for supporting patients with chronic diseases are vast. Once again, occupational therapy practitioners have been serving the community with chronic disease for decades. However, they are not a staple among the care team when it comes to palliative care. Only approximately 14% of people with chronic illness who need palliative care currently receive it, and the global need for palliative care will continue to trend upward because of the aging population and the impact of noncommunicable and some communicable diseases (World Health Organization, 2020). At this rate, there are not enough palliative care providers to support the number of patients facing chronic illness. Practitioners can help in these efforts by providing patients with education and skilled services to help manage disease symptoms and promote independence in daily life.

Summary

Occupational therapy's ability to assess the person, environment, and occupation and then execute an individualized treatment plan to promote independence is an authentic part of its DNA. Occupational therapy and palliative care share a similar goal of helping patients improve their QoL through management of a chronic disease or illness. Ultimately, occupational therapy and palliative care share the belief that greater support lends itself to greater care. Those facing chronic illness deserve the very best care, and a model such as palliative care affords them this right.

Lindsey Buddelmeyer, OTD, MOT, OTR/L, is the Leadership Education & Training Specialist at Blanchard Valley Health System in Findlay, Ohio. She has a personal and professional passion for advocating and working with the chronic disease community. Previously, she has worked as a full-time faculty member at the University of Findlay, and as an adjunct for St. Catherine University in their postprofessional doctorate program. Lindsey also worked as an occupational therapist on the palliative care team for 4 years. She has also served as a consultant and continues her work with the Ohio Council for Cognitive Health. Lindsey has been published and presented at the state and national level during the past 10 years of her career. These experiences and platforms have included a wide range of community and professional organizations involving topics surrounding chronic illness, palliative, and hospice care.

Andrea Sensel, OTD, OTR/L, is an occupational therapist with 15 years of experience who has passionately served older adults in multiple settings for the majority of her career. Currently, Andrea is the Doctoral Capstone Coordinator and Assistant Professor of Occupational Therapy at the University of Findlay in Findlay, Ohio. Current research interests include older adult fall prevention, successful aging in place, and effectiveness of home modifications. In addition to teaching and sharing her passion for serving older adults with her students, Andrea enjoys continuing to educate older adults through community-based programming, which include CarFit, Stepping On, and Tai Chi for Arthritis. Andrea is also a member of the Ohio Older Adults Fall Prevention Coalition and the Ohio Agency on Aging 3 Advisory Board.

REFERENCES

Ainsworth, E., & de Jonge, D. (2019). The home modification process. In E. Ainsworth & D. de Jonge (Eds.), *An occupational therapist's guide to home modifications* (2nd ed., pp. 83–110). Slack.

Alzheimer's Association. (2022). *Help and support*. https://www.alz.org/help-support

American Occupational Therapy Association. (2015a). *Occupational therapy's role with chronic disease management*. https://www.aota.org/-/media/corporate/files/aboutot/professionals/whatisot/hw/facts/factsheet_chronicdiseasemanagement.pdf

American Occupational Therapy Association. (2015b). *The role of occupational therapy in palliative and hospice care.* https://www.aota.org/~/media/Corporate/Files/AboutOT/Professionals/WhatIsOT/PA/Facts/FactSheet_PalliativeCare.pdf

American Occupational Therapy Association. (2020). Occupational therapy practice framework: Domain and process (4th ed.). *American Journal of Occupational Therapy, 74*(Suppl. 2), 7412410010. http://doi.org/10.5014/ajot.2020.74S2001

Bhatnagar, S., & Patel, A. (2018). Effectiveness of the certificate course in essentials of palliative care program on the knowledge in palliative care among the participants: A cross-sectional interventional study. *Indian Journal of Palliative Care, 24,* 86–92. https://pubmed.ncbi.nlm.nih.gov/29440814/

Cai, C., & Hu, J. (2016). Effectiveness of a family-based diabetes self-management educational intervention for Chinese adults with type 2 diabetes in Wuhan, China. *Diabetes Educator, 42,* 697–711. https://doi.org/10.1177/0145721716674325

Center to Advance Palliative Care. (2020). *The case for community-based palliative care.* https://www.capc.org/documents/download/867/

Eva, G., & Morgan, D. (2018). Mapping the scope of occupational therapy practice in palliative care: A European Association for Palliative Care cross-sectional survey. *Palliative Medicine, 32,* 960–968. https://doi.org/10.1177/0269216318758928

Granbom, M., Taei, A., & Ekstam, L. (2017). Cohabitants' perspective on housing adaptations: A piece of the puzzle. *Scandinavian Journal of Caring Sciences, 31,* 805–813. https://doi.org/10.1111/scs.12400

Gunten, C. (2012). Evolution and effectiveness of palliative care. *American Journal of Geriatric Psychiatry, 20,* 291–297. https://doi.org/10.1097/JGP.0b013e3182436219

Habitat for Humanity. (2022). *Frequently asked questions.* https://www.habitat.org/about/faq

Harris, J. R., & Wallace, R. B. (2012). The Institute of Medicine's new report on living well with chronic illness. *Prevention of Chronic Disease, 9,* 120126. https://doi.org/10.5888/pcd9.120126

Javens, C. (2021). *Palliative care: What can I bill?* https://www.axxess.com/blog/financial/palliative-care-what-can-i-bill/

Jefferson Elder Care. (2022). *Professional training: Skills2Care.* https://www.jefferson.edu/academics/colleges-schools-institutes/rehabilitation-sciences/jefferson-elder-care/professional-training.html

Koketsu, J. (2018). Activities of daily living. In H. Pendleton & W. Schultz-Krohn (Eds.), *Pedretti's occupational therapy: Practice skills for physical dysfunction* (8th ed., pp. 155–229). Elsevier.

Mackichan, F., Adamson, J., & Gooberman-Hill, R. (2013). "Living within your limits": Activity restriction in older people experiencing chronic pain. *Age and Ageing, 42,* 702–708. https://doi.org/10.1093/ageing/aft119

Mathiowetz, V., Finlayson, M., Matuska, K., Chen, H., & Luo, P. (2005). Randomized controlled trial of an energy conservation course for persons with multiple sclerosis. *Multiple Sclerosis, 11*, 592–601. https://doi.org/10.1191/1352458505ms1198oa

Milazzo, S., Hansen, E., Carozza, D., & Case, A. (2020). How effective is palliative care in improving patient outcomes? *Current Treatment Options in Oncology, 21*(12). https://doi.org/10.1007/s11864-020-0702-x

Mthembu, T., Brown, Z., Cupido, A., Razack, G., & Wassung, D. (2016). Family caregivers' perceptions and experiences regarding caring for older adults with chronic disease. *South African Journal of Occupational Therapy, 46*, 83–88. http://www.scielo.org.za/scielo.php?script=sci_arttext&pid=S2310-38332016000100015

Nasreddine, Z., Phillips, N., Bedirian, V., Charbonneau, S., Whitehead, V., Collin, I., . . . Chertkow, H. (2005). The Montreal Cognitive Assessment, MoCA: A brief screening tool for mild cognitive impairment. *Journal of the American Geriatrics Society, 53*, 695–699. https://pubmed.ncbi.nlm.nih.gov/15817019/

National Academics of Sciences, Engineering, and Medicine. (2016). *Families caring for an aging America*. The National Academics Press. http://doi.org/10.17226/23606

Ornstein, K. A., Aldridge, M. D., Mair, C. A., Gorges, R., Siu, A. L., & Kelley, A. S. (2016). Spousal characteristics and older adults' hospice use: Understanding disparities in end-of-life care. *Journal of Palliative Medicine, 19*(5), 509–515. https://doi.org/10.1089/jpm.2015.0399

Parkinson's Foundation. (2022). *Resources and support*. https://www.parkinson.org/Living-with-Parkinsons/Resources-and-Support

Reisberg, B. (1988). Functional Assessment Staging (FAST). *Psychopharmacology Bulletin, 24*, 653–659.

Sabbagh, M. N., Silverberg, N., Bircea, S., Majeed, B., Samant, S., Caviness, J. N., Reisberg, B., & Adler, C. H. (2005). Is the functional decline of Parkinson's disease similar to the functional decline of Alzheimer's disease? *Parkinsonism & Related Disorders, 11*(5), 311–315.

Sclan, S., & Reisberg, B. (1992). Functional Assessment Staging (FAST) in Alzheimer's Disease: Reliability, validity, and ordinality. *International Psychogeriatrics, 4*, 55–69. https://doi.org/10.1017/S1041610292001157

Stark, S., Keglovits, M., Somerville, E., Ling-Hu, Y., Barker, A., Sykora, D., & Yan, Y. (2021). Home hazard removal to reduce falls among community-dwelling older adults: A randomized clinical trial. *JAMA Network Open, 4*(8), e2122044. https://doi.org/10.1001/jamanetworkopen.2021.22044

Stark, S., Somerville, E., & Russell-Thomas, D. (2011). Choosing assessments. In M. Christenson, & C. Chase (Eds.), *Occupational therapy and home modification: Promoting safety and supporting participation* (pp. 25–43). AOTA Press.

Strong, S., & Rebeiro Gruhl, K. (2011). Person–environment–occupation model. In C. Brown & V. C. Stoffel (Eds.), *Occupational therapy in mental health: A vision for participation* (pp. 46–31). F. A. Davis.

Szanton, S., Leff, B., Li, Q., Breysse, J., Spoelstra, S., Kell, J., . . . Gitlin, L. (2021). CAPABLE program improves disability in multiple randomized trials. *Journal of the American Geriatric Society, 69,* 3631–3640. https://agsjournals.onlinelibrary.wiley.com/doi/full/10.1111/jgs.17383

The Hartford. (2022). *At the crossroads: Family conversations about Alzheimer's disease, dementia & driving.* https://s0.hfdstatic.com/sites/the_hartford/files/cmme-crossroads.pdf

Wingardh, A., Goransson, C., Larsson, S., Slinde, F., & Vanfleteren, L. (2020). Effectiveness of energy conservation techniques in patients with COPD. *Respiration, 99,* 409–416. https://doi.org/10.1159/000506816

World Health Organization. (2020). *Palliative care.* https://www.who.int/news-room/fact-sheets/detail/palliative-care

World Health Organization. (2022). *Palliative care: Essential facts.* https://www.who.int/multi-media/details/palliative-care---essential-facts

Yu, J., Yap, P., & Liew, T. M. (2018). The optimal short version of the Zarit Burden Interview for dementia caregivers: Diagnostic utility and externally validated cutoffs. *Aging and Mental Health, 23*(6), 706–710. https://doi.org/10.1080/13607863.2018.1450841

Zemke, R., & Clark, F. (1996). *Occupational science: An evolving discipline.* F. A. Davis.

6

Delivering Occupational Therapy Services in Hospice Care

DAVID BENTHALL, MS, OTR/L, and HEATHER McKAY, PhD, OTR/L

Learning Objectives

After completing this chapter, readers will be able to

- explain the purpose of occupational therapy in end-of-life care;
- identify common care challenges faced by patients and families in hospice;
- describe occupation-based practice models that foreground occupational participation at the end of life;
- describe Medicare hospice guidelines that support occupational therapy services for patients at the end of life;
- differentiate occupational therapy intervention approaches aligned with the hospice philosophy from traditional rehabilitative approaches;
- specify types of interventions that enable occupation at the end of life and promote quality of life for hospice patients and their families; and
- analyze the occupational therapy process in the context of a hospice case example, including assessments, goals, interventions, and outcomes guided by the *Occupational Therapy Practice Framework*.

Key Terms and Concepts

- adaptation-based approach
- advocacy
- caregiver training
- discharge
- Doing–Being–Becoming framework
- durable medical equipment
- end-of-life occupations
- energy conservation
- evaluation process
- home modifications
- hospice
- intervention approach
- intervention implementation
- intervention plan
- intervention review
- legacy building
- Medicare hospice benefit
- occupational participation
- occupational profile
- outcomes
- person–environment fit
- plan of care
- relaxation techniques
- symptom management

Occupational therapy practitioners provide skilled, occupation-centered care to patients and their caregivers throughout the lifespan, including the end of life. People nearing the end of life are eligible for ***hospice,*** a comprehensive patient- and family[1]-centered care model focused on quality of life (QoL) in the final stage of a disease that includes occupational therapy services. Historically, occupational therapy services have predominantly been situated in traditional biomedical models of practice in which rehabilitation potential and goals to optimize independence drive the patient's plan of care. However, occupational therapy's focus shifts away from independent performance when a patient is terminally ill and functional declines are expected.

The overarching purpose of occupational therapy in hospice is to improve QoL for patients and families by facilitating meaningful occupational participation despite the patient's declining functional abilities. Occupational therapy practitioners offer a distinct occupational perspective on well-being at the end of life that is theory driven, research informed, and aligned with the hospice philosophy that all people deserve compassionate care in the last phases of incurable disease so that they may live as fully and comfortably as possible. Despite a patient's diagnosis, condition, or time remaining, practitioners recognize that having opportunities to participate in meaningful occupations remains vital for

[1] In this chapter, the term *family* includes blood relatives, friends, informal caregivers, or anyone identified by the patient as being in their inner circle.

health, wellness, and QoL throughout a person's life course. Thus, occupational therapy promotes living life to the fullest all the way to the end of life by enabling positive occupational experiences that improve QoL and well-being for everyone involved in the dying process (American Occupational Therapy Association [AOTA], 2016).

Building on the important history and evidence justifying occupational therapy in hospice detailed in Chapter 4, "Hospice and Occupational Therapy," this chapter provides a practical guide for occupational therapy practitioners working in hospice and for students and practitioners interested in exploring this challenging and rewarding practice area. This chapter also provides resources for other stakeholders (e.g., hospice agencies, interdisciplinary team members, consumers) who want to know what to expect from occupational therapy practitioners in end-of-life care.

This chapter begins by exploring common care challenges and the benefits of ***occupational participation*** for patients and families at the end of life. We offer an occupation-based practice model that reframes the intent of therapy and foregrounds occupation's benefits despite the patient's expected functional decline. Next, the chapter explains how patients are referred to occupational therapy in hospice. Then, using the *Occupational Therapy Practice Framework: Domain and Process* (4th ed.; *OTPF–4;* AOTA, 2020) as a road map, we trace the occupational therapist's steps through assessment, intervention planning, implementation, and discharge. Along the way, we address common how-to questions and share practice tips to satisfy those who wonder what enabling occupation looks like and what are desired, achievable outcomes for patients who are simultaneously living and dying. Throughout the chapter, readers are guided through the story of a patient named James and his spouse Nancy to connect knowledge and skills to a real-world example of occupational therapy in hospice care (see Case Example 6.1).

Common Care Challenges for Hospice Patients and Families

Hospice is an approach to care that focuses on a person's comfort and QoL as they approach the end of life. It is important to remember that hospice is a subsection of palliative care designated for people experiencing life-limiting illnesses for whom curative measures are no longer desired

CASE EXAMPLE 6.1. INTRODUCING JAMES

James was a 66-year-old man with Stage 3 lung cancer who was admitted to his local Veterans Health Administration medical center after developing pneumonia and back pain that had been worsening over the past 2 weeks. James had been battling Stage 3 lung cancer for the past 2 years with the support of his spouse, Nancy. Despite the aggressive nature of James's cancer, he described himself as a fighter throughout this process and endured months of chemotherapy and radiation to battle the disease.

While James was hospitalized, his inpatient oncology team immediately got to work to further examine his symptoms and underlying causes of his change in medical status. To better assess James's functional level, he was referred to occupational therapy for evaluation and treatment and to provide safety recommendations for discharge. The inpatient occupational therapy assessment revealed important clinical information regarding James's level of function. Before the hospitalization, James's baseline level of function 1 month earlier was seemingly stable. Despite the challenging symptoms associated with chemotherapy treatments, James was modified–independent with self-care performance and mobility in the home because he required increased time to complete daily living tasks as a result of shortness of breath.

In contrast, the inpatient occupational therapist assessed James as being significantly below his prior level of function. As a result of pneumonia, James's breathing was more labored in comparison with baseline, and he required continuous oxygen (3 liters/minute) to maintain normal oxygen saturation levels. He exhibited significant limitations in mobility as evidenced by needing maximum assistance to perform basic bed mobility and was unable to sit at the edge of bed for longer than 2 minutes because of back pain. He also required up to maximum assistance in performance of self-care, with most of his ADLs being performed at bedside because of dyspnea symptoms. James's immediate goal was to regain adequate strength so that he could return home while independently managing his self-care. He expressed that he did not want to place any more burden on his wife.

The occupational therapist worked with James once a day during his inpatient hospitalization while his pneumonia was treated. The goals of treatment included improved independence in self-care and functional mobility needed for a successful transition home. The therapist used a variety of interventions to improve James's independence, including ADL retraining to increase his self-care performance, transfer training from hospital bed to wheelchair to optimize strength, seating and positioning strategies to manage pain, and energy conservation

(Continued)

CASE EXAMPLE 6.1. INTRODUCING JAMES *(Cont.)*

strategies to manage underlying fatigue and shortness of breath. However, very limited progress toward these rehabilitative goals was documented; James was unable to tolerate treatments because of his level of fatigue and breathlessness. James's level of dyspnea directly affected his participation in therapy sessions to the point where he needed rest breaks for very simple functional activities such as brushing his teeth and rolling in bed.

After undergoing several tests while in the hospital, James received the unfortunate news from his oncology team that despite best efforts, his cancer was no longer responding to treatment. There was evidence that James's lung cancer had metastasized to several organs in his body, including his spine, which explained his severe back pain. After 10 days in the hospital, James bravely expressed to his wife, Nancy, that he was finished with the battle to beat cancer and wanted to transition home to spend his remaining time where he was most comfortable. Despite his fighter mentality, James accepted the news of his prognosis and talked with his oncology team about forgoing further life-sustaining treatments. This prompted the team to facilitate a difficult conversation about goals of care with James and Nancy who, after much consideration, agreed that their desires were for comfort-based care as opposed to curative care and accepted a referral for hospice services.

or appropriate (Hospice Foundation of America, 2018). Hospice and palliative care both aim to optimize QoL and relieve challenging symptoms for people with serious illnesses; however, hospice is a specialized service focusing on comprehensive comfort care for people with a life expectancy of 6 months or less and includes support for families.

Within hospice care, there is a strong focus on managing problematic symptoms that are associated with the dying process to support a person's QoL at the end of life. Care challenges vary on the basis of a person's illness, but commonly cited symptoms for people in hospice care include difficulty with pain management, lack of energy, fatigue, shortness of breath, poor appetite, and difficulty sleeping (Connor, 2018a). Families frequently experience their own challenges adjusting to the responsibilities of their evolving role. Family responsibilities can include managing their loved ones' physical and emotional care, medications, household, and financial needs while simultaneously trying to balance their own personal care and engagement in meaningful occupations (Keesing & Rosenwax, 2011).

In addition to challenging physical symptoms, people approaching the end of life and their families may also experience emotional, social, and spiritual challenges as they cope with the dying process. A person in hospice care may be grieving multiple losses as they approach death, including the loss of being a healthy person, of being able to work, of being able to care for oneself, and of family and friends and the anticipatory grief of dying (Connor, 2018b). Hospice services help alleviate these symptoms through a holistic and interdisciplinary approach that places the patient's and family's needs at the center of treatment. As noted in Chapter 4, there is strong evidence that hospice services are effective in helping patients and their families manage problematic symptoms as patients approach the end of life. However, research has suggested that many hospice patients and families still have unidentified or unresolved occupational concerns leading up to and immediately after the person's death.

Occupation at the End of Life

As a person approaches the end of life, engaging in valued occupations may become increasingly difficult over time as a person loses functional independence (Bye, 1998). Declines in occupational performance may be associated with physical pain; motor, sensory, or cognitive decline; and emotional distress, and the person may require increased caregiver support to accommodate these challenges at the end of life (AOTA, 2016). Persons with a terminal illness can also experience a significant disruption in their previously established roles and routines. Not being able to participate in daily life and meaningful occupations as one desires can contribute to the loss of self-identity, loss of control, disengagement from daily life, social isolation, and, ultimately, occupational deprivation (Keesing & Rosenwax, 2011). Living with a terminal illness can also affect the ability to maintain valued social relationships (Chow, 2018).

Despite the negative aspects of a life-limiting illness, it is important to note that approaching death does not mean a person loses their desire to live. In fact, the importance of engaging in everyday occupations may be heightened and more meaningful for people who are approaching the end of life (Jacques & Hasselkus, 2004). Consider the importance of engaging in familiar, everyday routines such as preparing a morning cup of coffee or enjoying a favorite meal with family. These daily occupations may become even more important to patients and families as they navigate their end-of-life journey and try to preserve the familiar routines of everyday life (la Cour et al., 2009; Peoples et al., 2017).

In addition to ways that people continue with daily life, people approaching the end of life also consider ways to prepare for death. This may result in shifting priorities to occupations that are most important to the patient and family, including spending time together with loved ones, saying goodbye, and getting personal affairs in order (Chow & Pickens, 2020). Occupational therapy practitioners recognize that having the opportunity to engage in meaningful occupations at the end of life supports health, well-being, and QoL (AOTA, 2017, 2020). The ability to participate in meaningful occupations based on their desires and interests is an option that all people should have (Marcil, 2006).

Addressing the unmet occupational needs of patients and families in hospice care presents opportunities for occupational therapy practitioners to be key players on the hospice team. The goal of occupational therapy services in end-of-life care is not rehabilitation or returning a patient to a higher level of independence. Instead, practitioners in hospice use an ***adaptation-based approach*** that meets patients and their families where they are in their end-of-life journey and adjust interventions to optimize occupational participation as patients approach death. This approach allows practitioners to focus on a person's QoL and, specifically, how a person and family choose to engage in occupations that are most important to them despite functional declines. An adaptation-based approach includes a dual focus on supporting patients in their goals to continue life while also preparing for death (AOTA, 2016).

To better align with the goals and philosophy of hospice, occupational therapy practitioners must embrace the principles of palliative care that optimize patients' QoL while simultaneously reducing suffering. Pizzi (2015) described this concept as a shift from an illness trajectory to a wellness trajectory in which practitioners can support patients' ability to participate in life to their fullest potential. With a renewed focus on occupational participation and QoL, practitioners can help maximize patients' remaining abilities to engage in occupations that are most important to them and in the environment in which they want to participate (AOTA, 2016; Chow, Pickens, Fletcher, Thompson, et al., 2022; WFOT, 2016).

Occupation-Based Practice Models Appropriate for End of Life

Occupational therapy practitioners help facilitate patients' engagement in meaningful occupation throughout the entire life course, including at the end of life. Although people at the end of life are expected to experience progressive loss of function, approaching death does not preclude a person from achieving a sense of health or wellness (Lyons et al., 2002). Wilcock (1998) claimed that health and wellness can be achieved at all stages of life by having the opportunity to engage in valued occupations. This view of health and wellness is less influenced by a person's medical diagnosis or level of function or dysfunction than by their available opportunities, access, and support to engage in meaningful occupations (i.e., lack of opportunities, access, or support leads to occupational deprivation, alienation, imbalance, and injustice). By understanding patients as occupational beings, practitioners can ground their perspective in the core belief that occupation is transactionally related to health and well-being and has the power to facilitate a good death experience for everyone involved in the dying process (AOTA, 2016; Jacques & Hasselkus, 2004; Pizzi, 2010).

Wilcock (1998) stated that occupational therapy practitioners should embrace an understanding of occupation that "includes all the things that people do, the relationship of what they do to who they are as human beings, and that through occupation they are in a constant state of becoming different" (p. 248). This understanding of occupation is referred to as the ***Doing–Being–Becoming framework.*** This framework illustrates that occupational engagement is not only about doing at certain times but that it also has the transformative potential to help people discover themselves and achieve growth and self-actualization throughout the life course regardless of dysfunction, illness, disability, or time remaining. This transformative view of occupation at the end of life (i.e., that participation in meaningful occupations can be made not only possible but also health supporting for everyone involved in the dying process) contrasts significantly with common views of aging and dying, which are mostly symbolized by images of loss, decline, and incapacity to engage in daily life (Lyons et al., 2002).

Too often, patients with a life-limiting illness may be perceived as not needing or qualifying for occupational therapy services on the basis of their condition or limited life expectancy (a misperception based on a restrictive, disease-focused rehabilitative model; Chow, Pickens, Fletcher, Bower, et al., 2022). However, when occupational therapy practitioners apply an occupation-based perspective (change their lens) to look beyond a dying person's illness or rehabilitative potential and focus more on their potential to engage in their own life with the people closest to them, they can more readily see occupation's impact on QoL as a person nears the end; recognize opportunities, supports, and barriers; and facilitate adaptation and continued occupational participation for patients and families involved in the dying process (Benthall & Holmes, 2011; Chow, Pickens, Fletcher, Bower, et al., 2022).

The Doing–Being–Becoming framework is useful to understand people's occupational potential throughout the life course, including the final stage, and it can help occupational therapy practitioners demonstrate and explain occupational therapy's value in end-of-life care, expanding practitioners' collaborative role with (extending their professional reach to) more people living with a terminal illness and the hospice teams who support them. Case Example 6.2 reintroduces James as he enters hospice care and explores his personal goals and desires to continue life despite declining function.

Occupational Therapy Referrals in Hospice

A referral for occupational therapy services can be generated at any point in hospice care to address a patient's occupational needs and goals. The ***Medicare hospice benefit*** includes the provision of occupational therapy services for patients receiving hospice to help address symptom management and to help enable ADLs and basic functional skills (Centers for Medicare & Medicaid Services [CMS], 2021). When there is a skilled and medically necessary need for occupational therapy services that coincides with the hospice philosophy of care, patients receiving hospice have the right to access these services.

Occupational therapy services delivered in hospice must be provided under a physician's written order or prescription in the patient's medical record. However, a referral for occupational therapy can be initiated by multiple sources, including the patient and family caregiver,

CASE EXAMPLE 6.2. JAMES: BEGINNING HOSPICE SERVICES

At his request, James was discharged from the hospital back to his home under hospice services, which began immediately. Services included regular visits by his hospice nurse, social worker, chaplain, and personal care aide, who visited intermittently throughout the week to offer support and provide end-of-life care to James and Nancy. Over time, the regular in-home visits fostered a trusting partnership with the hospice team as James and Nancy navigated this unexpected and challenging journey.

The hospice team set James up in a hospital bed in his bedroom, which was at the rear of his single-level home. James remained in his hospital bed full time, and he required dependent-level care for ADLs and basic bed mobility. He required continuous oxygen (3 liters/minute) for palliative management of dyspnea symptoms and to help him remain comfortable. A primary goal of treatment was to optimize pain control for James's back, which was most relieved via pharmacological management and when he was in a semi-reclined position in bed. James's dependent level of care meant that his spouse Nancy was the primary family caregiver, managing the heavy-duty lifting, rolling, and positioning to assist James with his self-care goals. The physical strain of managing James's care added to the mental stress she was experiencing in accepting James's declining functional status and the fact that he was nearing the end of life.

James's level of function changed dramatically. In the course of 1 month, he shifted from being active and engaged in his daily life while managing cancer to being totally bedbound. Television was the only thing James felt as though he had control over, and the social isolation started to affect his overall QoL and well-being. In one of his weekly meetings with his hospice nurse, James said, "I just wish I could get out of bed and do something that made life worth living. I hate lying here all the time feeling like I can't do anything. Even if it's for a short amount of time, I wish I could spend a little time out of bed with my family." Despite limitations that included pain and shortness of breath, James indicated that he still had a desire to participate in life. He just did not know how to do it. The hospice nurse listened to James's wishes and shared this information with the hospice interdisciplinary team during their weekly patient care meeting. After discussion, the team recommended a hospice occupational therapy referral to evaluate James on the basis of his identified occupational concerns.

the occupational therapy practitioner, and other hospice interdisciplinary team members (i.e., physicians, nurses, social workers, counselors, chaplains, other rehabilitation therapists). Patients and families who are able to self-advocate and identify their own challenges may request services, such as occupational therapy, through their hospice case manager. This is dependent on the patient's and family's previous knowledge and awareness of occupational therapy services. Alternatively, referrals for occupational therapy services may be initiated by interdisciplinary team members. Although many hospice team members may not fully understand the role of occupational therapy in end-of-life care, it is critical to advocate and educate team members about occupational therapy's distinct value in hospice. This allows team members who have more frequent contact with patients and families to better identify patients who could benefit from occupational therapy services. Expanding team members' awareness on occupational therapy's role in hospice can optimize appropriate and timely referrals so that patients and families can receive occupational therapy services at the right time and in the right way (Chow, Pickens, Fletcher, Bower, et al., 2022). Educating referral sources on occupational therapy's role can also mitigate the risk of inappropriate referrals.

In addition to providing education to hospice team members, interdisciplinary team meetings can be an excellent venue for promoting occupational therapy services. Hospice interdisciplinary teams must meet at least every 15 days to review and revise a patient's individualized care plan. The frequency of interdisciplinary team collaboration provides a perfect opportunity for education and advocacy. In meetings, occupational therapy practitioners listen for patients' and families' occupational concerns and needs that are not being fully addressed, challenges that limit patients' participation in meaningful occupational roles and routines, performance deficits, and environmental supports and barriers.

For example, imagine a nurse in a team meeting reporting that a patient with advanced Parkinson's disease is struggling with self-feeding and is becoming more reliant on their spouse for meals. This could be an immediate cue for an occupational therapy practitioner to inquire further about those challenges (e.g., "Does self-feeding difficulty interfere with the patient's or family's QoL?" "Is optimizing participation in mealtime routines a patient or family goal?" "Have strategies previously been tried to address the occupational challenge, and what were the results?").

Engaging in dialogue with team members in interdisciplinary meetings can generate more appropriate and timely occupational therapy referrals. Listening, asking questions, and advocating for occupational therapy involvement in a team meeting can be critically important to getting a foot in the door and spreading awareness about the positive impacts occupational therapy practitioners can have when working with patients and families in hospice care.

Occupational Therapy Assessment and Goals of Care

The evaluation process is the first opportunity for the occupational therapist to become familiar with the patient and family in hospice care and attempt to understand their priorities and goals. According to the *OTPF–4,* the ***evaluation process*** "is focused on finding out what the client wants and needs to do; determining what the client can do and has done; and identifying supports and barriers to health, well-being, and participation" (AOTA, 2020, p. 21). For the patient approaching the end of life, the evaluation process is grounded in their occupational needs and ways to facilitate participation in meaningful occupations to enhance QoL in their remaining time. Given the fluctuating nature of the patient's medical condition as well as their illness trajectory, the evaluation process must be highly adaptive to the patient's changing situation, and assessment should be ongoing. Therapists must also be attuned to the needs of families and other caregivers and incorporate their perspective during the evaluation.

OCCUPATIONAL PROFILE

Just as in any other practice setting, the occupational therapy evaluation of a hospice patient begins with the creation of an ***occupational profile*** (AOTA, 2020). Creating an occupational profile enables the practitioner to more fully understand who the patient is as a person, the ways in which the patient desires to participate more fully in life, and perceived supports and barriers that are affecting participation in their chosen meaningful occupations. The occupational profile establishes a narrative that recognizes the patient in hospice care as a person with interests, values, priorities, and goals that are not limited by illness or life expectancy.

Investing time in the occupational profile for the patient at the end of life can be even more meaningful because it fosters a process of life review and further affirms the patient as an occupational being with ongoing desires and ambitions. It also provides insight into the patient's outlook on life and their beliefs about and expectations of the dying process (AOTA, 2016). When possible, the evaluation process also includes investigation of the family's and other caregivers' experiences and the ways in which the occupational therapist can support them in fulfilling their roles. This is particularly important when the patient is less able to express their desires and wishes related to their care (Cooper & Kite, 2015). The occupational profile establishes a partnership with the patient and family in which goals can be determined collaboratively to ensure the treatment plan is patient and family centered.

INTERVIEWS, OBSERVATIONS, AND ASSESSMENT INSTRUMENTS

Interviews and observations of the patient and caregiver in the context of their environment are fundamental during the evaluation process to identify the occupations that are still relevant and meaningful to the patient (Cooper & Kite, 2015; Pizzi, 2015). A qualitative study of occupational therapists working in hospice overwhelmingly cited their use of interviews and observations, as opposed to formal, standardized assessments, as primary assessment methods used with patients and their identified care partners (Bye, 1998). Because of the extremely personal and emotional nature of experiences surrounding death and dying, working with patients in hospice requires a strong foundation in patient-centered care and in therapeutic use of self to help identify what matters most to the patient during their last phase of life (Pizzi, 2015). This means that the therapist must remain present, authentic, and aware of personal judgments and biases during the evaluation process (Pizzi, 2010). Therapists use effective communication skills that enhance collaborative problem solving and cooperation with patients and families, such as active listening, affirming the patient's wishes, and formulating explanations and suggestions that are patient and family centered and contextually relevant.

In interviews with the patient and family, occupational therapists use open-ended questions to gather meaningful, qualitative responses that target the patient's self-perceptions of their end-of-life care goals. This includes an examination of a patient's cultural, spiritual, and social factors

(AOTA, 2016). Keeping in mind that the hospice patient is approaching their last phase of life, occupational therapists should ask patients open-ended, occupation-centered questions, such as "What is most important for you to do? Experience? Finish? Remember? Pass along? Say?" The patient should be allowed time to process and formulate responses at their level of comfort and insight into their condition. In these critical, caring conversations, patients and families need time and space to respond, so it is important for the therapists to exercise patience and become comfortable during times of silence instead of overtalking, understanding that there may not be an easy answer or an immediate solution. Responses to interview questions can provide meaningful information about the patient's underlying motivations and goals while further directing analysis of occupational participation. Listening behaviors can be used in hospice to reframe, restate, and reflect information yielded in the clinical interview to allow the patient to hear their own words and to also clarify the therapist's understanding of what the patient and family are conveying (Davis et al., 2013). Using a skilled interview and observation of the patient in hospice can optimize patient-centered care and establish the occupational therapy plan of care in the occupations that are most meaningful to the patient and family members.

Evaluation methods may vary depending on the patient's needs and whether use of formal or standardized assessments is clinically indicated. Although standardized measures can yield relevant information, it is important to note that there are no established or accepted occupational therapy outcome measures or assessments specific to hospice care (Chow, 2018). Chow and Pickens (2020) conducted a scoping review of the occupational therapy literature that revealed a paucity of occupation-based outcome measures with psychometric strength and clinical utility that specifically measure occupational participation, consider environmental contexts, and explore specific end-of-life occupations.

Because there are no hospice-specific occupational therapy instruments, assessments frequently used in end-of-life care include the Canadian Occupational Performance Measure (COPM; Law et al., 2019), Occupational Circumstances Assessment Interview and Rating Scale (OCAIRS; Forsyth et al., 2005), Goal Attainment Scaling (GAS; Kiresuk & Sherman, 1968; Kiresuk et al., 2014), Pizzi Holistic Wellness Assessment (Pizzi, 2001), Functional Assessment of Chronic Illness Therapy–Spiritual Well-Being Scale (Cella et al., 1993; Noguchi et al., 2004), and

Self-Efficacy Scale for Terminal Cancer (Hirai et al., 2002). The Relative Mastery Scale (RMS; George-Paschal et al., 2022) is another potentially useful instrument for occupational therapists working in hospice. Based on the theoretical perspective of occupational adaptation, the RMS identifies occupational challenges chosen by the patient; guides collaborative problem solving targeting the patient's adaptive process; and measures effectiveness, efficiency, and satisfaction with adaptive responses in the care environment from the perspective of the patient and others—a rare example of an instrument that captures perspectives of teammates working together (McKay, 2019).

Occupational therapists working in hospice should be aware that using strictly performance-based measures such as the FIM®, Barthel Index, or Katz Index of Independence in Activities of Daily Living may not capture change or progress toward occupational participation goals because these measures track the patient's performance skills, which are expected to decline over time in hospice care (Chow, 2018). Further research to establish outcome measures that reflect occupational therapy's skill set in hospice is needed. Thus, therapists should use their clinical reasoning skills to determine the best approach for each hospice patient by using assessment tools as needed, in conjunction with interviews and observation, to effectively gather relevant information on patient and family needs.

Fundamental to the occupational therapy evaluation is consideration of a patient's desire and ability to participate more fully in their daily life and meaningful occupations (i.e., what is most important to the patient?). The assessment should include an exploration of the patient's remaining physical, emotional, cognitive, and social abilities; the demands of the environment; and an analysis of the occupations that are important to the patient, and it requires an understanding of how the patient's terminal illness is disrupting or limiting engagement in daily life. For example, a patient with end-stage chronic obstructive pulmonary disease (COPD) may experience a functional decline in ADL performance associated with their illness. This patient may prioritize spending time out of bed using their available energy to share a daily meal with family instead of working on basic self-care skills. Alternatively, another patient with Stage 4 cancer with bone metastases might want to preserve their ability to access the bathtub because taking a warm bath improves their pain management and QoL. Although the patient in hospice may experience declining functional abilities over time, the role of the occupational therapy practitioner is to identify what is most important to the patient in the context of their end-of-life experience and consider ways to support continued participation in meaningful occupations by assessing the patient's strengths, capacities, and contexts (AOTA, 2016). The evaluation may also consider the family's skillset in delivering care and role competence to meet the patient's changing care demands.

After eliciting the patient's and family's priorities, it is important to evaluate supports and barriers in the patient's environment. Occupational therapy practitioners are most frequently referred for patients in hospice care who still reside in their home or natural environment. Observation of the home setting is critically important to understand the environmental barriers that are affecting participation in occupations. When possible, the occupational therapist should ask to tour the home environment. Touring the home environment allows the therapist to specifically observe the context in which performance occurs and to better understand strengths and barriers of the home environment (Siebert, 2016b).

When considering occupational participation as opposed to independent performance, occupational therapists can reflect on key questions (Chow, 2018): Can the patient's or family's roles or routines be modified to allow for continued participation in a meaningful occupation? Can the patient or family participate in a role or an occupation without performing an actual skill? Can a new occupation or role be introduced that is meaningful to the patient or family? Answering these questions can help broaden the therapist's perspective on ways in which they can address a person's participation in daily life that is less directed by occupational performance skills and more focused on holistic ways a person can engage in life on their terms and on the basis of their abilities.

PLAN OF CARE

Information yielded from the evaluation process helps the occupational therapist develop the occupational therapy ***plan of care.*** Patient-centered goals are created that reflect the occupations most important to the patient and family. Creating goals that are both meaningful and realistic is important for a person with limited life expectancy and requires communication and collaboration between the therapist and patient (Bye, 1998). Despite the patient's predictable functional declines, the therapist can still develop occupation-based goals that are specific, measurable, achievable, realistic, and timely. Instead of focusing on increasing independence, occupational therapy goals can target the patient's participation in occupation by grading the task to the patient's functional abilities, identifying cueing needs, and pinpointing environmental supports needed for the patient and caregiver to be successful.

Consider the following scenario of a patient in hospice who enjoys the occupation of bird watching. As a result of progressive weakness and functional losses, the patient spends all of her time in bed. From the bed, she cannot see her favorite bird feeder outside the window, so she is disengaged from a preferred leisure activity that historically reduced her stress and boredom. An objective goal for this patient could be written as follows: "Within 2 weeks, caregivers will complete 3 environmental modifications to the bedroom to facilitate the patient participating in her preferred leisure occupation, bird watching, to decrease social isolation." This goal is occupation based and measurable, has an established time frame, and describes what action will lead to accomplishment of the end objective. With a focus on enabling occupational participation to improve QoL, the goal demonstrates a way to incorporate environmental modifications and caregiver involvement in the plan of care. Creating meaningful goals should also reflect role competence in families and their ability to safely manage the patient's care at the end of life.

FREQUENCY

Decisions about how often to see a patient and family in hospice and for how long should be determined by medical necessity as well as the trajectory of the patient's functional status. The trajectory of a patient's condition may be hard to predict in hospice, but occupational therapists should integrate their knowledge of the patient's past performance with their knowledge of the patient's current condition to envision their visit frequency (Siebert, 2016a). The duration of services should also be grounded in the skilled needs of the patient and family caregivers. For example, a therapist might find that one patient's goals will be met in one or two visits, whereas another patient may benefit from skilled occupational therapy services multiple times for several weeks to reach their goals. A determination of the frequency and duration of occupational therapy services is made in collaboration with the patient and family and should be considered skilled, medically necessary, and aligned with the hospice philosophy on the basis of the patient's identified goals. Hospice interdisciplinary team meetings and other communication with team members yield useful data that contribute to the occupational therapy plan of care.

Once the occupational therapy goals, proposed interventions, and frequency and duration of visits are determined, the occupational therapy plan of care is documented in the patient's medical record and submitted to the hospice physician for approval and concurrence. Using these patient-centered and occupation-based approaches to evaluation, occupational therapists can better support a person approaching death to achieve a more positive end-of-life experience (see Case Example 6.3).

CASE EXAMPLE 6.3. JAMES: EVALUATION

During the evaluation, the occupational therapist understood that James's biggest goal was to do something meaningful out of bed. However, further exploration was needed to better understand who James was as a person and his occupational goals and motivations. The therapist was able to do this by completing an occupational profile. During the interview and observation of James, the therapist learned that James was previously independent in all aspects of his life and was quite active in his community before being diagnosed with lung cancer. James and Nancy had been married for 35 years, and they shared a daughter and two small grandchildren. He worked at his local paper mill and was nearing retirement before stepping down prematurely because of his diagnosis. As a veteran, James was a member of the local Veterans of Foreign Wars, which met monthly. He also served his community every week at a local food pantry, preparing meals for those in need. James loved to cook and shared this occupation with Nancy. Nancy confirmed that food was an important part of their family culture and that cooking was one of their favorite ways to spend time together. Since coming home, James reported that cooking was a role and routine that he had to pass over to his wife.

After better understanding James and his valued occupations, the occupational therapist shifted the interview to problem solve James's goals. The therapist specifically asked James to describe what would be most meaningful for him to do if he was able to spend time outside of his hospital bed. Responding to guided and open-ended questions, James was able to elaborate, stating, "I just don't feel very connected to my family. I feel stuck back here in my bedroom and

(Continued)

CASE EXAMPLE 6.3. JAMES: EVALUATION *(Cont.)*

I can't do anything." Underscoring James's desire for greater connectedness with his family, he stated, "I would love to get out of this room and enjoy a meal with my wife. I would love to cook again. I would love to visit with my daughter and grandchildren. These are all things we take for granted, but I wish I could just do something." The therapist asked what he thought the barriers were to participation out of bed, and James expressed, "I can't sit for long at all due to my pain. We tried sitting up on the edge of bed in the hospital, but I couldn't tolerate it. The only position I feel comfortable in is when I'm reclined in bed. When my pain gets bad, my breathing gets bad, too." This was demonstrated by moving James's upper body through different positions using the electric hospital bed. When positioned in sitting at 100 degrees hip flexion, James expressed severe pain. However, James indicated adequate pain relief when lowered back to 120 degrees. James then expressed, "I don't think there's much hope. I need to just accept this is my life now and get used to it."

The occupational therapist used empathy to reflect both James's challenges and his hopes and goals for the time that he had remaining. Using therapeutic use of self, the therapist expressed a desire and willingness to work together with James and Nancy to accomplish James's end-of-life goals by taking a step-by-step approach to determine his tolerance for activity while also exploring different sitting and positioning mechanisms that could optimize his pain control out of bed. James and Nancy were both willing to try and agreed to work with the therapist to determine any possible solutions.

In comparison with James's goals in acute care, which focused on improved independence in self-care and mobility, James's goals in hospice shifted toward participation in the activities that were most meaningful to him and directly influenced by the nature of his terminal illness. All of James's goals were connected to his desire to continue living life despite his limitations.

Occupational Therapy Intervention

Once the occupational therapy evaluation is complete, it is time to consider the patient's intervention plan. The occupational therapy ***intervention plan*** guides intervention and is based on a synthesis of information yielded from the occupational profile, analysis of occupational performance, and patient and family goals that directly guide treatment (AOTA, 2020). Siebert (2016a) described the intervention plan as a "road map for the journey the occupational therapy practitioner and the patient will take together" (p. 99). In consideration of the patient's end-of-life care goals, it is critical that the interventions delivered in hospice be patient centered and developed in collaboration with patients and their families, as evidenced by interventions being meaningful and guided by the patient's goals and wishes. Interventions should enable the patient and family caregiving team to maintain as much engagement as possible in occupations that are related to their life roles. Such engagement best occurs when interventions are adaptable, tailored to fit patient and family caregiver capabilities, and consider activity and environmental demands that influence participation in daily life (AOTA, 2016).

APPROACH

Interventions delivered by the occupational therapy practitioner in hospice are not unlike interventions delivered in traditional practice settings. What is different in hospice is how the ***intervention approach*** is applied. Interventions in hospice focus on enabling patients to participate in daily life in the ways they choose despite declining functional abilities and with assistance from family and other caregivers as needed. The decision to foreground occupation and participation while deemphasizing pathology, performance skills, and independence is intentional. Regaining independence or resuming a higher level of function may not be possible or realistic as a person approaches the end of life. By shifting the focus to engaging together with others, the ultimate aim of every intervention approach is enhanced QoL for the patient and family in the patient's remaining time. Thus, using only a remediation or traditional rehabilitative approach to practice is not recommended because it does not coincide with the hospice philosophy of care, described in Chapter 4. A closer look at intervention approaches can help therapy practitioners and other stakeholders appreciate what is different about occupational therapy in hospice and what remains consistent with practice in other areas.

The *OTPF–4* identifies five approaches that direct the intervention process: health promotion, remediation, maintenance, modification, and prevention (AOTA, 2020). Occupational therapy practitioners often use more than one intervention approach when working toward a patient goal or specific outcome (Siebert, 2016a). When considering a patient's trajectory in hospice care, one might expect the patient to have experienced a progressive decline in function associated with a terminal or chronic condition. Thus, occupational therapy interventions appropriate in hospice might be less focused on remediation as used in traditional rehabilitation settings and more focused on promoting occupational participation for as long as possible by modifying activity and environmental demands, maintaining engagement in occupations and roles that are important to the patient, and preventing injury to the patient and identified family caregivers. The combination of these approaches in hospice helps to preserve the patient's and family's participation in meaningful occupations while minimizing any performance or environmental barriers that may exist.

IMPLEMENTATION

After carefully considering the intervention plan and approach, it is time to deliver the intervention, otherwise known as ***intervention implementation.*** Interventions in hospice most frequently occur face to face and in the context of the patient's home. However, occupational therapy practitioners might consider supplementing home visits with telephone calls or other telemediated encounters to monitor progress toward goals, provide caregiver support and education, and reinforce recommendations made during a previous occupational therapy visit (Siebert, 2016a). Although interventions in hospice are not unlike interventions delivered in other practice areas, occupational therapy practitioners working in hospice settings have a dual focus on maximizing occupational engagement in the moment to continue living while simultaneously delivering interventions that help patients and families prepare for death (Chow, 2018). Practitioners specifically address end-of-life occupations that are most meaningful to the patient and their family that promote life review and help achieve closure to promote a good death (Pizzi, 2010). Practitioners can also direct interventions to reduce negative symptoms that may be affecting function. ***Symptom management*** could include care to relieve pain, shortness of breath, fatigue, anxiety, fear, and depression. Interventions in hospice should not only be directed toward the patient but also consider the essential role of families and other caregivers during the dying process. These interventions are explored in further detail in the "End-of-Life Occupations and Activities" section.

REVIEW

It is also important to note that depending on the duration of intervention and how quickly the patient's disease is progressing, changes may be observed in the patient's body functions, such as muscle, sensory, and mental functions, and interventions and goals may have to be adapted accordingly. This process is called ***intervention review,*** which requires occupational therapy practitioners to continually review intervention delivery and progress toward goals (AOTA, 2020). If changes are noted in the patient's functional status, practitioners should adjust the interventions accordingly using grading techniques, which could include further adapting the task or environment. Progress toward occupational therapy goals can be documented despite a patient experiencing functional decline as long as the goals of care are targeted toward occupational participation as opposed to independent performance. However, unanticipated circumstances may result in changes that prompt the practitioner to consider the need to continue or discontinue occupational therapy services (Siebert, 2016a).

End-of-Life Occupations and Activities

Supporting a patient with a terminal condition to participate more fully in life during the dying process can be just as if not more important to the patient in the last phase of life. ***End-of-life occupations*** are specific and meaningful activities that may be unfamiliar to the patient, be unique to the dying process, and influence and shape a person's end-of-life experience (Jacques & Hasselkus, 2004). Patients approaching the end of life may shift their focus toward occupations such as prioritizing important relationships, seeking closure, saying goodbye, engaging in legacy building and life review, adjusting life to accommodate illness, divesting themselves of valued objects, and putting final affairs in order (Bye, 1998; Chow & Pickens, 2020; Hunter, 2008b; Jacques & Hasselkus, 2004; la Cour et al., 2009; Marcoux, 2001). The importance of these end-of-life occupations may be heightened for a patient with a terminal illness and require the occupational therapy practitioner to shift their approach and incorporate interventions that meet the patient's occupational needs.

In a scoping review investigating occupational therapy's efficacy in end-of-life care, researchers Chow and Pickens (2020) found that occupational therapy practitioners had a disproportionate focus on occupational performance as opposed to occupational participation in end-of-life care and mostly practiced in an "ADL–IADL box" (p. 7). This focus represents a missed opportunity for practitioners to address patients' specific occupational needs shaped by the dying process. Interventions may vary in hospice depending on what is most important to the patient and family. However, a practitioner might incorporate several interventions when working with patients in hospice care that address end-of-life occupations and help patients and families to prepare for death.

One intervention strategy an occupational therapy practitioner may use with patients involves the construct of ***legacy building.*** The transmission of legacy is described by Hunter (2008a) as a way in which people make meaning of life through "the process of passing oneself through generations, creating continuity from the past through the present to the future" (p. 314). Legacy building uses life review to identify the core spirit of who a person is, including their key values, beliefs, accomplishments, and life lessons. In its most basic form, legacy building is a narrative for how a person wants to be remembered. A practitioner engaging in legacy building might consider how patient narratives can be transmitted in different ways, including storytelling, autobiographies, recordings, traditions, pictures, and objects of importance. For example, a practitioner working with a patient at the end of life could incorporate photographs as a form of storytelling to engage the patient in life review. A practitioner might consider ways for a patient to write letters to their grandchildren or document the patient's stories virtually (e.g., recording, videotaping) so that the patient's narratives are passed on to loved ones. These stories have the potential to support the patient in finding closure, reconnecting with loved ones, strengthening relationships, and also saying goodbye. Passing along narratives honors the patient's life and can add meaning to the end-of-life process.

Divesting themselves of valued possessions and determining where important objects will go after death is also a common consideration for people with a terminal illness (Peoples et al., 2018). Marcoux (2001) described this process of divesting oneself of objects of importance as a construction of the self through emptying of the home. Whether an heirloom piece of jewelry or a used set of farm tools, objects accumulated over time have the power to symbolize history, tradition, meaning, and personal value. The meaning attached to cherished objects incorporates a person's life narrative, has the potential to continue after death, and can be representative of a person's legacy (Hunter, 2008a). The occupational therapy practitioner working with a patient in hospice should be aware of objects of importance and consider ways to incorporate those items and narratives in the intervention process. For example, an occupational therapy intervention could include helping a patient document a traditional family recipe to give to their family, ensuring that an important family custom is maintained. Practitioners can also engage patients in therapeutic activities to facilitate the expression of creativity. Bye (1998) found that many patients in hospice had a desire to create gifts as a way to leave something concrete and tangible to their loved ones after their death. Creative expressions can symbolize a way for patients to have closure in the dying process and give patients choice, control, and the ability to make decisions about how they want to be remembered (Peoples et al., 2018). This process of divesting themselves of objects can also help identify and incorporate people of importance into the practitioner's intervention with the patient.

Supporting Everyday Occupations to Continue Daily Life

In addition to helping patients prepare for death, occupational therapy services can also support patients to continue valued roles and routines of daily life. Research has indicated that people living with a life-limiting illness desire to continue living and maintaining engagement in their usual occupations (Jacques & Hasselkus, 2004; la Cour et al., 2005, 2009; Peoples et al., 2017). Bye (1998) described this concept of maintaining everyday routines as an attempt to create a sense of normality for people in hospice care (p. 13). Jacques and Hasselkus (2004) found that approaching the end of life brought new meaning to and appreciation of the ordinary and familiar occupations of daily life for patients in hospice, including maintaining life roles, routines, and social relationships. Occupational therapy practitioners can assist patients in hospice to maintain participation in desired life roles and occupations by recognizing that having the opportunity to participate in daily life contributes to QoL as well as to cope with the dying process (AOTA, 2016).

To help support a patient in hospice to continue daily life, an occupational therapy practitioner can consider ways to adapt tasks and environments so that the patient can still perform meaningful occupations. By assessing the patient's strengths and barriers in the context of the environment, the practitioner may problem solve ways in which the patient can adjust life to accommodate illness. For example, a patient with end-stage COPD living in a long-term-care facility desires to maintain participation in a weekly dominos game with friends that has become an important tradition and social support for the patient. However, management of fatigue as well as transporting the oxygen tank has become too burdensome. The practitioner may analyze the task and environment and identify ways to facilitate this meaningful activity in a way that meets the patient's needs. Examples could include determining times of the day when the patient feels strongest, exploring strategies for transporting oxygen to conserve energy, or inviting the patient's friends to her primary living environment to reduce unnecessary energy expenditure with management of oxygen. Even at an advanced stage of disease, the practitioner might consider ways the patient can participate and be involved in this meaningful dominos game through observation to facilitate social connection. Making minor adjustments to the task and environment provides the patient with greater support to continue this valued occupation and minimizes the risk of social isolation even as the disease progresses.

Another example is a new mother who has terminal Stage 4 breast cancer. As a result of lymphedema, the patient is struggling to hold and feed her newborn because of pain in her affected extremity and fatigue. Given the importance of the patient's role as a mother, an occupational therapy practitioner could explore adaptations such as wraps or slings to support the patient in holding her child while minimizing the physical burden. The practitioner could also explore the patient's social support systems and ways she can participate in mothering occupations with support from her partner, family, or friends.

These examples represent how a person might want to continue life despite illness and the ways in which an occupational therapy practitioner might use their skill set to help a patient prioritize relationships of importance and engagement in meaningful occupations despite illness. By facilitating the patient's participation, the practitioner honors the patient's wishes to engage in life and valued occupations in whatever capacity is possible, further optimizing a more positive end-of-life experience.

Reducing Negative Symptoms: Symptom Management

An aspect of achieving a good death for patients is through reducing negative symptoms such as pain, fatigue, breathlessness, and anxiety and maintaining comfort and control during the dying process (Pizzi, 2010). An occupational therapy practitioner working in hospice care must address the medical nature of a patient's condition and the ways in which the condition affects their participation in occupation. In the following sections, we discuss common strategies to address symptom management in hospice care.

PAIN MANAGEMENT

Occupational therapy practitioners may discover that a patient's barrier to participation in meaningful occupations is related to pain that they are experiencing near the end of life. For hospice patients, managing pain can include both pharmacological and nonpharmacological strategies and requires close consultation with the patient's medical team, including the hospice physician and nurse. Prescribing medications falls to physicians and nurse practitioners, but the practitioner may have valuable input regarding pain management strategies based on the patient's wishes and desired activity level. For example, a patient who wants to transfer out of bed each morning for breakfast or for a community outing may require strategic timing and dosing of medications. In that case, the practitioner would notice and report the effects of medicines, based on their understanding of the patient's pain in the context of their preferred activity, and collaborate with the hospice team, including the attending physician, to tailor a medication regimen that fits the capabilities of the patient and caregiver (AOTA, 2017).

Occupational therapy practitioners in hospice address habits and routines surrounding medication management, modify environments to make medication management easier and safer, and adapt the patient's preferred activities to optimize participation with as little pain as possible. The practitioner may also reinforce education related to medication organization and administration as determined by the physician and alert the hospice team and physician to any negative effects of medications on occupational performance (AOTA, 2017).

The occupational therapy practitioner may be more involved and focused on nonpharmacological pain management interventions with patients at the end of life. Training can be provided in the use of physical agent modalities, such as heat or ice, gentle exercises such as stretching and range of motion, breathing exercises, relaxation strategies, positioning techniques, proper body mechanics, guided imagery, and pacing activities. Pain management strategies or modalities can be used before, during, or after engagement in activity to manage symptoms to the patient's satisfaction. Nonpharmacological pain management strategies may vary on the basis of the person's condition and their occupational goals. Careful understanding of the patient and family using interview, observation, and pain assessments can help determine what type of nonpharmacological strategies they value and are willing to try or have worked for them in the past.

FATIGUE MANAGEMENT

Patients at the end of life may often experience diminished energy that affects their ability to engage in daily life. Occupational therapy practitioners should consider training in energy conservation strategies when the patient is experiencing symptoms such as pain, breathlessness, fatigue, or anxiety that interferes with participation in desired occupations. ***Energy conservation*** is a method of using specific strategies tailored to the patient that reduce the amount of energy expended when performing an activity. Using energy conservation complements an end-of-life care approach in occupational therapy because it targets ways to adapt activities, environments, and personal strategies to enable engagement.

When working in hospice care, the occupational therapy practitioner can help patients prioritize what activities are most important to them and determine which activities they would most like to conserve their energy to perform (Cooper & Kite, 2015). This process is 100% patient centered because it directs the patient and family to prioritize the occupations that are most important to them. Alternatively, the practitioner can help identify unnecessary or less valued tasks that might deplete energy resources and partner with a caregiver to lessen the burden of those tasks. For example, a person with multiple sclerosis and notable weakness might be willing to use an electric lift rather than self-transferring out of bed to save energy. By doing the activity in a different way or with assistance from a caregiver, the person can direct their energy toward the occupation that is most meaningful to them with minimal disruption.

Occupational therapy practitioners can assist patients with planning and organizing activities that match their functional capacity. Considerations can include thinking about times of the day that work best for the patient and spreading activities out over time to minimize fatigue. Other examples include pacing and identifying strategies to balance activity with opportunities for rest. Breathing techniques, such as pursed-lip breathing and diaphragmatic breathing, can also be implemented to help reduce fatigue or anxiety (American Lung Association, 2020; UC San Diego Health, 2021). The practitioner may consider environmental supports, equipment, and positioning strategies for the patient in hospice care to maximize their comfort when engaged in activity (Cooper & Kite, 2015).

Last, the occupational therapy practitioner's understanding of activity in the context of the environment and the patient's abilities and limitations can be an asset on a hospice team. In hospice care, patients or families may often have the perception that they cannot engage in activities because of their condition, prognosis, or limited functional capacity. The occupational therapy practitioner is vital in helping to recognize and problem solve strategies patients and families can use to enable participation in occupations that are most important to the patient. Practitioners help patients identify valued occupations while also giving them permission to disengage from activities that are not a priority (see Case Example 6.4).

CASE EXAMPLE 6.4. JAMES: INTERVENTION

Working with James two times a week for 8 weeks, the occupational therapist designed and implemented multiple interventions guided by James's desire to "get out of bed and do things that make life worth living." Keeping occupational participation as their main intent, James, his wife, and the occupational therapist devised strategies to manage pain, complete environmental modifications to make getting out of bed easier and safer for the couple, and make activity adjustments to reconnect James with chosen health-supporting occupations.

To compensate for James's low back pain issues, the occupational therapist started by evaluating seating and positioning strategies. The therapist determined that James's low back pain was most relieved when in a semireclined position (approximately 120 degrees hip flexion) and exacerbated when seated fully upright. Thus, the therapist recommended and prescribed a high-back reclining wheelchair to allow James to fully customize his seated experience and allow him to change positions while out of bed to relieve pressure on his lower back. Instead of working on manual transfers, the therapist recommended an electric lift that would support participation in out-of-bed transfers with minimal physical exertion so

(Continued)

CASE EXAMPLE 6.4. JAMES: INTERVENTION *(Cont.)*

that James could save his energy and direct it toward his activity goals. This involved coordination with the hospice interdisciplinary team as well as the contracted durable medical equipment vendor to complete the equipment requests using James's Medicare hospice benefit. After accessing the wheelchair and electric lift in the home, the therapist worked with James and Nancy to safely transfer James out of bed while incorporating pursed-lip breathing technique to reduce anxiety and dyspnea. The first time James successfully transferred to the wheelchair using the lift, Nancy was brought to tears, stating, "I never thought I'd see you out of bed again." James was also filled with emotion and enjoyed navigating outside to get fresh air for the first time in a month. The therapist was able to adjust James's seating and positioning using the wheelchair mechanics to minimize his pain level. This allowed James to remain out of bed for 60 minutes with acceptable pain control.

The occupational therapist worked with James and Nancy over several sessions to problem solve safe transfer strategies using the electric lift as well as wheelchair seating and positioning needs to maximize James's pain management while out of bed. After James and Nancy demonstrated greater confidence with management of transfers, the therapist was able to transition the intervention toward his meal preparation goals—a core occupation for James and his wife. Because cooking was a valued co-occupation that allowed James and Nancy to spend time together, the therapist shared an unconventional idea to modify the space in the breakfast nook to fit James's hospital bed. The kitchen was literally and figuratively the center of the home. This would pull James out of his bedroom and allow him to feel more connected to his family, including his daughter and grandchildren when they come to visit. Positioning James in proximity to the kitchen would also allow the couple to spend time together while Nancy cooked, something they both enjoyed. To James, watching and visiting during meal preparation made him feel more engaged in the activity even if he was not physically performing the task. James and Nancy were both satisfied with the new arrangement and the environmental modifications, which immediately started to lift James's spirits.

Given that James was able to tolerate at least 60 minutes out of bed, the occupational therapist worked collaboratively with James and his wife in the kitchen to modify a workspace so that James could assist in meal preparation tasks in a semi-reclined position. The therapist problem-solved strategies to adapt meal preparation so that James could participate at his level of comfort with Nancy's

(Continued)

CASE EXAMPLE 6.4. JAMES: INTERVENTION *(Cont.)*

support. For example, when making a pot of soup, James was able to stir and monitor the soup from a comfortable wheelchair position while Nancy performed some of the more complex tasks, such as preparing and chopping the vegetables. James was also able to participate in a cooking session with his grandchildren, teaching them how to make a loaf of sourdough bread. Using a lap tray on his wheelchair, James and his grandchildren were able to roll and form dough together as a meaningful activity while Nancy supervised and assisted as needed. The therapist also incorporated adaptive equipment, including nonskid mats and utensils with built-up handles to compensate for James's weakened grip. By modifying the environment and adapting the task, James was able to participate at his level of comfort or transition to a more observational role. This further enhanced the activity of cooking as a co-occupation between James, Nancy, and their grandchildren.

To address ongoing symptoms of dyspnea, fatigue, and pain related to James's cancer diagnosis, the occupational therapist infused energy conservation strategies throughout the interventions to include mindfulness, self-pacing, deep breathing, and incorporation of rest breaks as needed to minimize negative symptoms. Using these strategies along with proper wheelchair seating and positioning, James was eventually able to tolerate 2 hours of out-of-bed activity. This was long enough for James to enjoy a meal that he helped make for the first time in months at the dinner table with his wife, daughter, and grandchildren as opposed to eating meals in his hospital bed.

Given that food was such an important aspect of James's family culture, the occupational therapist engaged him in several interactions centered around food and meal preparation that facilitated a sense of life review. Reminiscing led James to describe stories of how his mother taught him to cook at a young age. James told stories of working in the kitchen while overseas during the Vietnam War. He also described special family recipes and traditions that had been passed down within his family that were meaningful to him. James's stories opened the door for the therapist to approach the concept of legacy building. The therapist candidly asked James during a visit, "How do you want to be remembered by your family?" "Are there items you want to pass down to your family?" and "Are there goals that you want to accomplish with your time remaining?" In a difficult yet honest conversation about death, James spoke intently about his desire to consolidate important family recipes that were important to him in his life and pass them

(Continued)

CASE EXAMPLE 6.4. JAMES: INTERVENTION *(Cont.)*

along to his family. James had always had this goal in the back of his mind but had assumed he had sufficient time remaining to complete it before his cancer diagnosis.

Because food and cooking were such a large part of James's life, the occupational therapist supported James in writing down several favorite recipes that were important to him and assembling them into a simple recipe book. In addition to consolidating the recipes, the therapist facilitated a video recording session in which James shared specific family memories that were attached to these recipes as a way for his family to share his legacy long after James died. This end-of-life occupation developed into a very meaningful project that gave James purpose during this last phase of life when managing the unfortunate symptoms of cancer were becoming more challenging. Although cooking was an important part of living, it was also an important aspect of preparing for death.

STRESS MANAGEMENT

People nearing the end of life may experience emotional distress that can affect their participation in daily life and meaningful occupations. In addition to physical pain, patients with a terminal illness may experience existential stress and anticipatory grief as they cope with the complex emotions that may accompany the dying process. When addressing stress management in hospice, an occupational therapy practitioner can use several different techniques that can help patients achieve greater comfort, control, and QoL. However, it is important to note that people cope with stress and grief in different ways. Thus, any strategies explored must be patient centered and within the patient's and caregiver's level of comfort.

One method occupational therapy practitioners might use when addressing stress management is relaxation techniques. ***Relaxation techniques*** include guided imagery, progressive muscle relaxation, movement therapies (e.g., yoga, tai chi), aromatherapy, and breathing techniques (i.e., diaphragmatic breathing). Using relaxation techniques incorporates all of a person's senses and creates a greater connection between mind, body, and spirit to help cope with stress. These strategies can support the patient to decrease overall muscle tension that may be present as a result of physical pain as well as biopsychosocial stressors (Collins et al., 2022). Relaxation techniques can be incorporated before, during, and after participation in an activity to help promote a patient's awareness and mindfulness of their thoughts, feelings, and sensations when engaged in a meaningful occupation. Practitioners can lead patients and families in performing relaxation techniques during intervention sessions but should also teach patients how to incorporate preferred techniques into their roles and routines to help cope with the stressors associated with death and dying.

Education and Training

Families play an integral role on the hospice team and provide a significant amount of physical and emotional support to their loved one as they approach the last stage of life. Friends and neighbors can also be informal caregivers. This network of family and friends may collaborate with additional paid helpers who contribute to the patient's care. Assuming the role of caregiver for a person nearing the end of life comes with many challenges and often lacks a road map or easy answers. However, most informal caregivers typically have limited experience in providing care for a terminally ill person (Connor, 2018a).

In occupational therapy, the terms *client* and *patient* are inclusive of both the person receiving hospice care and the family caregivers involved in the patient's care (AOTA, 2020). This is consistent with the hospice philosophy of care that treats the patient and family as the collective unit of care (Pickens & Long, 2016; Pizzi, 2015). Thus, it is critically important to fully incorporate identified family members in the occupational therapy plan of care to address their needs through caregiver training and support them in fulfilling their roles.

Families may fulfill a range of roles when assisting a loved one in hospice care, including providing direct care, assisting with decision making and goal setting, and honoring a patient's wishes through advanced care planning (Glajchen, 2016). Families are often expected to assist in many aspects of the patient's medical care, such as with medications, personal care, skin integrity, dressing changes, pain control, catheter care, oral care, and use of supplemental oxygen (Connor, 2018a). The needs of family members may, at times, exceed those of the person in hospice care; thus, hospice team members may need to identify supports to aid family caregivers in fulfilling their assumed role (AOTA, 2016).

Caregiver training may take on different forms in hospice care to address a family member's physical, social, psychological, and spiritual needs (Glajchen, 2016). When supporting a loved one in hospice, the family must adapt and respond to ongoing disease progression. As the patient experiences functional decline, the caregiver must adjust their level of support in response to the patient's limitations. This may not always be intuitive to family members or paid caregivers and may require the skills of an occupational therapy practitioner to address. Training may involve working with the family or other caregivers to identify their own personal strengths and barriers that affect care of the patient, problem solving to adapt the task and environment to minimize caregiver burden, and helping to facilitate positive communication between the patient and caregiver.

Occupational therapy practitioners may work with identified caregivers in a variety of ways depending on the occupational concern. Practitioners may work with family members to grade physical assistance during tasks that support the patient's participation while maintaining their autonomy and dignity. A practitioner might frame activities as a co-occupation between the patient and caregiver, which allows the caregiver to "do with" as opposed to "doing for" the patient. This requires skilled observation of patient and caregiver interests and goals. A practitioner might work with families to modify the physical environment and incorporate adaptive equipment to improve safety and reduce caregiver burden. Training in the use of items such as ADL equipment, wheelchairs, transfer devices, pressure relief aids, and hospital beds might be more common in hospice care. Caregiver training might include strategies for range of motion, edema control, positioning, and body mechanics to assist with reducing negative symptoms and making the patient more comfortable. What may be perceived as simple strategies, such as adjusting the height of the hospital bed, using proper body mechanics, or identifying best methods for repositioning the patient in bed, could be groundbreaking to the caregiver who is carrying increased stress.

In addition, occupational therapy practitioners can be instrumental in facilitating collaborative problem solving among family members and paid caregivers, helping them adapt together and resolve their shared occupational challenges with teamwork. The importance of sharing such tips and demonstrating basic skills in the occupational context should not be underestimated.

Although the majority of this chapter has focused on patients who are able to verbalize their goals and needs, this may not always be the case for patients approaching the end of life. In these difficult situations, families are more heavily relied on to monitor for symptoms such as pain, dyspnea, anxiety, and restlessness. For example, a patient with advanced dementia may require occupational therapy intervention in hospice specifically for caregiver training to address dementia communication strategies, nonpharmacological strategies to reduce stress, or ADL needs, such as feeding. The combined needs of the patient and family may exceed family caregivers' capabilities, prompting consideration of long-term placement or transition to inpatient hospice care if the patient is approaching the final stages of life. The occupational therapy practitioner could be helpful in supporting that transition to best meet the patient's and family's needs in the context of changing environments and changing caregiver roles.

Last, family members may experience distress and suffering long after the patient has died, which also opens up opportunities for bereavement support and ways in which occupational therapy can support opportunities for family members to participate in occupations that foster healthy grieving and coping (AOTA, 2016).

Home Modification and Durable Medical Equipment

As a person in hospice experiences declining function, the physical environment may present new challenges for maintaining performance of daily routines and valued occupations (Chow, 2018). Occupational therapists are uniquely positioned to provide evaluation and intervention in the area of home modifications as well as the provision of adaptive equipment to promote patients' comfort, safety, and functional abilities as they near the end of life (Cooper & Kite, 2015). ***Home modifications*** are adaptations to the physical characteristics of the home environment that promote a person's function and safety in daily activities. Home modifications can range from simple to complex solutions, such as widening doorways, adding ramps, installing grab bars, setting up a raised toilet seat, or moving furniture to promote greater accessibility. Modifying the physical environment can allow for partial or full engagement in meaningful occupations, improve safety, and decrease caregiver burden (Chow, 2018). These modifications are most effective when there is optimal ***person–environment fit,*** which is defined as the degree to which a person's abilities match the characteristics of their environment. When working with a patient in hospice, the practitioner should tailor the environment in a way that maximizes patient and caregiver strengths, abilities, and preferences while decreasing limitations and barriers. Modifying the environment in a way that honors patient choice and preference can help facilitate both QoL and engagement in daily life.

Throughout the occupational therapy assessment and intervention, occupational therapy practitioners working in hospice respond to the patient's current needs and facilitate the patient's and family's adaptation to their current situation while anticipating their future needs on the basis of normal disease processes. Patients in hospice may experience quickly fluctuating or changing abilities. Thus, consistent reevaluation of environmental needs is recommended as patients and families adjust to the changing circumstances of their illness and end-of-life journey. Because of the temporal nature of hospice care and the limited life expectancy of patients, the occupational therapy practitioner's focus may be on the patient's immediate needs and making environmental adjustments that enhance usability. For example, consider a person who is in their final days of illness and wants to die at home, not in a hospital. A practitioner would work collaboratively with the patient and family as well as with external resources to determine more immediate environmental needs to accommodate the patient's dying wish. Making large-scale modifications such as remodeling may not be a viable option, depending on a patient's prognosis (Chow, 2018), but nonpermanent modifications to the environment or use of equipment that can be removed easily after a person's death can be effective (Bye, 1998). Sensitivity to the patient's condition and prognosis should be considered when making recommendations for equipment or home modifications.

Within hospice, ***durable medical equipment*** (DME) is a covered benefit under the Medicare hospice benefit guidelines. Covered DME in hospice care must be used to relieve pain or reduce disease severity, be directly related to managing the patient's terminal medical condition, or both (CMS, 2021). DME items may not be covered if they are determined to be unrelated to the patient's terminal condition. Occupational therapy practitioners may be involved in recommending DME in hospice as well as in providing training to patients and families in the correct use of these devices. Examples of DME a practitioner might recommend in hospice include, but are not limited to, hospital beds, wheelchairs, pressure-relieving devices, walkers, lifts, and ADL-related equipment. These devices may promote optimal positioning and comfort needed for engagement in meaningful occupations.

DME requires a physician's written order. Thus, occupational therapy practitioners should collaborate with the patient's hospice interdisciplinary team, hospice billing and coding team, and the hospice agency's contracted DME provider to help patients obtain the items they need. It may also be of value for practitioners to familiarize themselves with local vendors and lending closets in their area in the event the patient is not able to afford the equipment or insurance does not cover its cost. When properly recommended and utilized, DME can greatly influence a person's safety and facilitate participation in meaningful occupations in a way that promotes QoL. Alternatively, equipment that does not fit with the patient's and caregiver's capabilities can lead to frustration, misuse of equipment, and unintended financial consequence. Thus, the practitioner must carefully examine patient and caregiver abilities, understand the underlying barriers to occupational performance, and consider whether a piece of equipment or modification to the environment would effectively meet the family's needs.

Beyond the physical environment, occupational therapy practitioners can be involved in supporting a patient's and family's social, cultural, and spiritual environments at the end of life (AOTA, 2016). In hospice, this support can include working with patients and families to construct environments that minimize social isolation and facilitate access to favorite objects, people, and places that improve QoL (Chow, 2018), including giving patients and families choices about their environment and incorporating aspects of their occupational profile in creating a space that is filled with meaning and fosters dignity. Considerations can include access to meaningful pictures, religious symbols (if desired), favorite music, comforting smells, and nature to create a peaceful environment. It also includes having the space and opportunity to connect with loved ones on a spiritual level and to say goodbye.

Resources to Support Patients Nearing the End of Life and Their Families

Patients and families may experience immeasurable stress in dealing with issues related to death and dying. This time may be one of the most difficult life experiences for the patient and family. Without support from health care professionals, many families may not be able to find and access available community resources during this time. Thus, occupational therapy practitioners should be prepared to connect patients and families with timely resources that can help support them during their time of need and incorporate this education into their interventions. Hospice agencies may frequently use social work services to connect families with community resources because they may have greater breadth of knowledge regarding this area of practice. However, it does not preclude practitioners from providing families with education about resources to meet their unmet occupational needs. This education involves ***advocacy,*** which is a type of intervention practitioners use to empower patients to seek and obtain needed resources that can support health, well-being, and occupational participation (AOTA, 2020). Working in collaboration with other hospice disciplines is ideally recommended to reinforce needed education and support access to community resources.

Resources will vary from area to area depending on where patients are located. This requires occupational therapy practitioners to explore and be knowledgeable about resources that are available to best support their patients. Local resources may include Area Agencies on Aging, support groups, personal care agencies, respite services, adult day programs, transportation, and food-related resources. Families may benefit from education and support specific to their terminal condition. For example, the American Cancer Society, ALS Association, and Alzheimer's Association might be common resources for patients and families to obtain education specific to their condition and also connect with others virtually to facilitate a sense of belonging. Awareness of spiritual resources, such as chaplain services and bereavement counselors offered by hospice, can also be helpful for patients and families who are experiencing grief.

Even if occupational therapy practitioners are not employed by a hospice agency, those working in different health care environments can be helpful in connecting patients and families to their hospice benefit when the time is right. This requires clinicians to be able to distinguish differences in hospice and palliative care services; be knowledgeable of general hospice eligibility guidelines, including clinical and functional determinants; and be able to communicate clinical findings to patients, families, and interdisciplinary team members.

Occupational Therapy Outcomes

Outcomes are a fundamental aspect of the occupational therapy process and describe the results patients can achieve through occupational therapy intervention (AOTA, 2020). From the initial evaluation with the patient throughout the intervention process, the occupational therapy plan of care is ultimately directed by the patient's and family's desired outcomes related to occupational engagement. This requires occupational therapy practitioners to skillfully collaborate with patients and families and fully use therapeutic use of self to target outcomes that are meaningful as well as realistic and achievable. Within hospice care, outcomes are less focused on independent performance skills and more focused on the patient's and family's ability to participate in their desired occupations.

The *OTPF–4* (AOTA, 2020) indicates a variety of potential occupational therapy outcomes, including occupational performance, prevention, health and wellness, QoL, participation, role competence, well-being, and occupational justice. Even when considering patients who are approaching the end of life and experiencing declining functional abilities, any of these occupational therapy outcomes are possible when occupational therapy practitioners are focused on ways to support patients' and families' engagement in daily life and meaningful occupations. When describing occupational therapy outcomes for patients at the end of life, Bye (1998) stated that

> the outcome is not about independence or permanent rehabilitation to a normal life—hallmarks of traditional occupational therapy. It is about occupational therapists helping clients to realize their goals to connect with life, and people in their life, on a level beyond illness and receipt of care. Achieving this outcome affirms clients' lives. (p. 19)

Even when a patient's physical independence declines, occupational therapy practitioners can support patients to have greater control, choice, and autonomy over decision making that affects their daily routines and end-of-life preferences (Bye, 1998; see Case Example 6.5). This support includes recognition that authentic occupational participation can exist even through passive observation and is not solely based on physical engagement in a task (Peoples et al., 2018). For a person at the end of life, having the opportunity to engage in occupation at any level can make the difference in achieving a good death experience.

When considering specific outcome measures, occupational therapy practitioners must rely on their clinical reasoning skills to identify outcomes that are appropriate to the patient's functional status, the patient's stage in the dying process, and the family's needs (Chow, 2018). According

CASE EXAMPLE 6.5. JAMES: OUTCOMES

After 8 weeks working with James, the occupational therapy plan of care was concluded. During this time, the occupational therapist used their therapeutic use of self, patient centeredness, and occupation-based lens to focus James's plan of care on outcomes that were meaningful to him and his family. Participation in these occupations enhanced his QoL and was a positive outcome focused not on independence but on James's desire to live as fully as possible during his remaining time. Occupational outcomes included improved occupational participation, role competence, QoL, and well-being. Prevention was addressed as an outcome to reduce social isolation, and the patient's occupational justice was honored to facilitate opportunities for engagement in valued occupations at the end of life.

James passed away 30 days after the occupational therapy intervention was complete. During this time, James was able to spend time with his family in a meaningful way that allowed him to engage in the occupations that were most important to him during his last phase of life. He was not confined to his hospital bed in social isolation but was able to continue living on his terms, guided by his autonomy, choice, and dignity. This case example shows that occupational therapy services can be a powerful facilitator for occupational engagement at the end of life. James was not seen as silent, passive, or bedridden awaiting death, but as a person deserving of doing, being, and becoming through occupation. Using occupation as a therapeutic medium, James experienced growth and self-actualization even at the end of his life and was allowed to connect with his family on a level beyond illness. This allowed James and his family to engage in daily life on the basis of their desires and motivations while also experiencing closure during the dying process.

to a scoping review by Chow and Pickens (2020) on the efficacy of occupational therapy service in end-of-life care, there are no currently accepted occupational therapy outcome measures specific to hospice care. Patient-centered measures, such as the COPM and GAS, may be appropriate tools for use in palliative and end-of-care because they target collaborative goal setting and exploration of meaningful occupations for patients and families. However, very limited research exists that specifically tests the use of the COPM and GAS with the hospice population (Chow, 2018).

Although lack of occupational therapy–specific outcomes may certainly affect the profession's ability to advocate for its value in hospice, Chow and Pickens (2020) indicated that a person at the end of life can still experience outcome gains and improved occupational participation even if they have a decline in functional performance. Research in occupational therapy outcomes needs to further investigate patient-centered measures that may be more sensitive to capturing subtle changes in personal and meaningful outcomes at the end of life as opposed to a focus on performance-based measures (Chow, 2018). If only performance-based measures are used (e.g., Barthel Index, Katz Index of Independence in Activities of Daily Living, Lawton Instrumental Activities of Daily Living Scale, FIM, Palliative Performance Scale, Karnofsky Performance Scale), a patient in hospice may appear to achieve very limited progress toward goals because these common measures may not be sensitive enough to demonstrate a patient's progress toward goals as they approach the end of life and experience deteriorating functional skills over time (Chow, 2018).

Discharge

Achievement of desired outcomes may signify the end of occupational therapy services (Siebert, 2016c). ***Discharge*** from occupational therapy services in hospice may occur for a variety of reasons. Common examples of reasons for discharge are that the patient and family have met established goals, the occupational therapy intervention no longer results in measurable benefits, or the patient and family elect to discontinue services.

Discharge planning begins at the time of the initial evaluation and extends throughout the duration of the occupational therapy plan of care

(AOTA, 2020). This practice is no different in hospice care than in traditional occupational therapy practice settings. The discharge planning process helps guide the occupational therapy practitioner to reflect during each intervention session on whether the patient and family are making measurable gains in reaching their established goals. Even though practitioners may observe the patient physically or cognitively declining, this does not automatically mean they are not making progress toward goals and that occupational therapy services are no longer needed. The practitioner may adjust or modify the plan of care on the basis of changes in the patient's functional status, goals, or family needs. Although patients are nearing the end of life, they have greater opportunities to meet many of their goals if goals are written with participation, engagement, adaptations, and caregiver training in mind.

Documentation and Billing

The contents of the occupational therapy plan of care, including evaluation, intervention, outcomes, and discharge, must be documented in the patient's medical record under the written orders of the hospice physician. Occupational therapy services should be documented in a way that demonstrates the domain of occupational therapy and the strong clinical reasoning of the occupational therapy practitioner (Siebert, 2016b). This is important for advocacy of occupational therapy's role in hospice. Given that occupational therapy services are underused in hospice, clinical documentation is an important advocacy tool to demonstrate the profession's value and contributions to patients in this practice area. Clinical documentation includes face-to-face encounters, progress notes, and interdisciplinary team meeting huddles that become a part of the patient's medical record. Stakeholders, including other hospice disciplines, clinical supervisors, executive leadership, and payer sources, look to skilled documentation as one method to substantiate the need for and value of occupational therapy services. Thus, it is important to use this opportunity to advocate for the ways in which occupational therapy services promote positive outcomes for patients at the end of life. All documentation in the patient's medical record should be consistent with the operations of the hospice agency and Medicare guidelines, and it should also reflect skilled and medically necessary services provided by the practitioner.

To continue advocating for occupational therapy services for patients at the end of life, it is important to be knowledgeable of Medicare policies and guidelines that support occupational therapy practice for those with a life-limiting illness. A common myth exists in health care that skilled therapies such as occupational therapy are not reimbursable services for patients at the end of life if they are declining in function or unable to regain a higher level of independence. For example, if a terminally ill patient is no longer making progress toward traditional rehabilitation goals or does not exhibit the capacity to regain independence, an occupational therapist may feel pressure to discharge or not even recommend services beyond evaluation because of the patient's poor rehabilitation potential. These myths are not accurate and also not supported by the Medicare guidelines.

Occupational therapy practitioners work with a broad range of patients and people with conditions who may not return to permanent independence. In many of these circumstances, focusing on restoration or recovery of their lost physical functions is not practitioners' primary focus. Practitioners also consider adaptive approaches, compensatory strategies, adaptive equipment, DME, and environmental modifications to increase a person's function in their living environment. Even though the occupational therapy plan of care is not fully focused on recovery of lost physical skills, this does not mean that Medicare does not provide reimbursement for services.

The *Medicare Benefit Policy Manual* refers to rehabilitation services for patients with terminal conditions in Chapter 15, where it states that

> rehabilitative therapy may be needed, and improvement in a patient's condition may occur, even when a chronic, progressive, degenerative, or terminal condition exists. For example, a terminally ill patient may begin to exhibit self-care, mobility, and/or safety dependence requiring skilled therapy services. The fact that full or partial recovery is not possible does not necessarily mean that skilled therapy is not needed to improve the patient's condition or to maximize his/her functional abilities. The deciding factors are always whether the services are considered reasonable, effective treatments for the patient's condition and require the skills of a therapist, or whether they can be safely and effectively carried out by nonskilled personnel. (CMS, 2022, pp. 180–181)

In working with patients, occupational therapy practitioners may encounter situations in which achieving a higher level of independence is not a reasonable expectation. However, in those situations, we encourage practitioners to refocus their plan of care on a palliative approach that supports patients' goals to engage in the occupations that are most important to them. Whether serving patients in hospice or other practice areas, Medicare requires practitioners to consider whether the services provided are reasonable and necessary and whether performance of the essential intervention requires the skill set and qualifications of an occupational therapy practitioner (CMS, 2022). If an occupational therapy intervention can be carried out by nonskilled personnel and does not require the skills of an occupational therapy practitioner, then Medicare should not be billed.

The Medicare guidelines are also clear in the following statement: "While a beneficiary's particular medical condition is a valid factor in deciding if skilled therapy services are needed, a beneficiary's diagnosis or prognosis should never be the sole factor in deciding that a service is or is not skilled" (CMS, 2022, p. 178). Medicare guidelines are quite clear that occupational therapy practitioners cannot deny a person the right to services because they are approaching the end of life or have a terminal prognosis. Understanding patients' diagnosis and prognosis is important in deciding what approaches and intervention types to use, but practitioners cannot deny patients the opportunity to receive therapy because they have a life-limiting illness. Serving patients at the end of life recognizes that those living with a life-limiting illness have occupational rights to participate in everyday life and occupations despite prognosis or limited life expectancy (AOTA, 2020). Situations may arise in practice in which a person who is considered terminally ill or nearing the end of life may have unrealistic expectations regarding their prognosis or potential outcomes. This situation may not be uncommon, but practitioners are encouraged to always consider whether the requested services are considered reasonable and necessary and require the skill set of an occupational therapy practitioner.

Summary

Occupational therapy practitioners have a wealth of skills and strategies to offer patients in hospice care. Of highest importance, practitioners understand that despite disease, illness, or life expectancy, all people throughout the life course have the capacity to achieve well-being by engaging in occupations that are meaningful to them. Practitioners recognize that even at the end of life, patients have the ability to adapt, grow, evolve, and develop. Practitioners acknowledge that having access and opportunities to engage in occupations can help patients and families live the last chapter of life to the fullest and facilitate a good death experience.

The *OTPF–4* provides occupational therapy practitioners with a guide to the development and delivery of occupational therapy services focused on occupations that are most meaningful to the patient and family. However, it is important to recognize that occupational therapy in hospice is not intended to conform to a rehabilitative model of care. All services in hospice align with compassionate end-of-life care and acknowledge that as patients get closer to death, functional capacities are expected to decline. Thus, practitioners working in hospice adopt an adaptation-based approach, as opposed to a rehabilitation approach, to meet the evolving occupational needs of patients and their families, optimizing participation for QoL all the way to the end of life.

An adaptation-based approach means that occupational therapy interventions are designed to help the patient maintain, learn, and optimize functional skills as long as possible while simultaneously adjusting environmental modifications and activity demands as the patient needs more support. From this adaptation-based perspective, occupational therapy practitioners can focus equally on everyone involved in the dying process and design interventions to help families and other caregivers master the challenges related to their end-of-life roles and experiences. Emphasizing active, collaborative problem solving and adjusting plans as needs change, this approach allows patients and families to master current challenges, make the most of their remaining time together, and feel more prepared for future challenges while also grieving natural losses. Using this approach, practitioners can communicate and demonstrate the value of occupational therapy in a way that aligns with the hospice philosophy. Gaining a larger footing in this practice area will require ongoing advocacy and strong partnerships with stakeholders to meet the profession's potential in this emerging practice area.

David Benthall, MS, OTR/L, is an occupational therapist with a passion for serving older adult clients and caregivers in their homes and communities. David is currently working in Home Based Primary Care at the Durham VA Medical Center. He has previously worked in home health and hospice care settings and has served as an adjunct faculty member at the University of North Carolina at Chapel Hill's Division of Occupational Science and

Occupational Therapy. David has presented and published on the topic of occupational therapy in end-of-life care and advocacy in primary health care.

Heather McKay, PhD, OTR/L, is an occupational therapist, dementia care specialist, and international trainer and speaker on topics related to dementia care and caregiver education. She has more than 20 years of experience working with older adults and their myriad caregivers across various settings. Currently, she is the founder and manager of Partnerships for Health, a dementia consulting company providing education and support for professionals and families and consultation with organizations on dementia workforce development. In addition to her work in dementia care education, Heather enjoys teaching in the Division of Occupational Science and Occupational Therapy at the University of North Carolina at Chapel Hill, where she shares her experience and scholarship around productive aging, collective occupational adaptation, and occupational therapy in end-of-life care.

REFERENCES

American Lung Association. (2020, February 27). *Pursed lip breathing*. https://www.lung.org/lung-health-diseases/lung-disease-lookup/copd/patient-resources-and-videos/pursed-lip-breathing-video#:~:text=Pursed%20lip%20breathing%20helps%20control,can%20better%20control%20your%20breath

American Occupational Therapy Association. (2016). Role of occupational therapy in end-of-life care. *American Journal of Occupational Therapy, 70*(Suppl. 2), 7012410075. https://doi.org/10.5014/ajot.2016.706S17

American Occupational Therapy Association. (2017). Occupational therapy's role in medication management. *American Journal of Occupational Therapy, 71*(Suppl. 2), 7112410025. https://doi.org/10.5014/ajot.2017.716S02

American Occupational Therapy Association. (2020). Occupational therapy practice framework: Domain and process (4th ed.). *American Journal of Occupational Therapy, 74*(Suppl. 2), 7412410010. https://doi.org/10.5014/ajot.2020.74S2001.

Benthall, D., & Holmes, T. (2011). End-of-life care: Facilitating meaningful occupations. *OT Practice, 16*(9), 7–10.

Bye, R. (1998). When clients are dying: Occupational therapy perspectives. *Occupational Therapy Journal of Research, 18,* 3–24. https://doi.org/10.1177/153944929801800101

Cella, D. F., Tulsky, D. S., Gray, G., Sarafian, B., Linn, E., Bonomi, A., . . . Brannon, J. (1993). The Functional Assessment of Cancer Therapy scale: Development and validation of the general measure. *Journal of Clinical Oncology, 11,* 570–579. https://doi.org/10.1200/JCO.1993.11.3.570

Centers for Medicare & Medicaid Services. (2021). Coverage of hospice services under hospital insurance. In *Medicare benefit policy manual* (rev. 11056). https://www.cms.gov/manuals/Downloads/bp102c09.pdf

Centers for Medicare & Medicaid Services. (2022). Covered medical and other health services. In *Medicare benefit policy manual* (rev. 11288). https://www.cms.gov/Regulations-and-Guidance/Guidance/Manuals/Downloads/bp102c15.pdf

Chow, J. K. (2018). Occupational therapy in hospice and palliative care. In H. M. Pendleton & W. Schultz-Krohn (Eds.), *Pedretti's occupational therapy: Practice skills for physical dysfunction* (8th ed., pp. 1195–1213). Elsevier.

Chow, J. K., & Pickens, N. D. (2020). Measuring the efficacy of occupational therapy in end-of-life care: A scoping review. *American Journal of Occupational Therapy, 74,* 7401205020. https://doi.org/10.5014/ajot.2020.033340

Chow, J. K., Pickens, N. D., Fletcher, T., Bowyer, P., & Thompson, M. (2022). Missed opportunities to ease suffering: An explanatory model of occupational therapy utilization in end-of-life care. *American Journal of Hospice and Palliative Medicine,* 04990912211439. https://doi.org/10.1177/10499091221143917

Chow, J. K., Pickens, N. D., Fletcher, T., Thompson, M., & Bowyer, P. (2022). "You've got to do something": Developing occupational therapists' role in end-of-life care. *OTJR: Occupation, Participation, and Health, 43,* 109–118. https://doi.org/10.1177/15394492221088239

Collins, M. E., Ward, A. L., Breeden, K. L., & Rowe, N. (2022). Sensation, wounds, and pain. In A. J. Mahle & A. L. Ward (Eds.), *Adult physical conditions: Intervention strategies for occupational therapy assistants* (2nd ed., pp. 256–282). F. A. Davis.

Connor, S. R. (2018a). Symptom management and physical care. In S. R. Cooper (Ed.), *Hospice and palliative care: The essential guide* (3rd ed., pp. 43–59). Routledge.

Connor, S. R. (2018b). What are hospice and palliative care? In S. R. Cooper (Ed.), *Hospice and palliative care: The essential guide* (3rd ed., pp. 1–17). Routledge.

Cooper, J., & Kite, N. (2015). Occupational therapy in palliative care. In E. Cherny, M. Fallon, S. Kaasa, R. K. Portenoy, & D. C. Currow (Eds.), *Oxford textbook of palliative medicine* (pp. 177–183). Oxford University Press.

Davis, J., Asuncion, M., Rabello, J., Silangcruz, C., & van Dyk, E. (2013). A qualitative review of occupational therapists' listening behaviors and experiences when caring for patients in palliative or hospice care. *OTJR: Occupation, Participation and Health, 33*(1), 12–20. https://doi.org/10.3928/15394492-20121012-01

Forsyth, K., Deshpande, S., Kielhofner, G., Henriksson, C., Haglund, L., Olson, L., Skinner, S., & Kulkarni, S. (2005). *Occupational Circumstances Assessment Interview and Rating Scale (OCAIRS) Assessment Manual.* University of Illinois at Chicago.

George-Paschal, L., Krusen, N. E., & Fan, C. W. (2022). Psychometric evaluation of the Relative Mastery Scale: An occupational adaptation instrument. *OTJR: Occupation, Participation and Health, 42,* 154–161. https://doi.org/10.1177/15394492211060877

Glajchen, M. (2016). *Family caregivers in palliative care and hospice: Minimizing burden and maximizing support*. National Hospice and Palliative Care Organization. https://www.nhpco.org/wp-content/uploads/2019/04/PalliativeCare_Family_Caregivers.pdf

Hirai, K., Suzuki, Y., & Tsuneto, A. (2002). Development of a self-efficacy scale for terminally ill cancer patients. *Japanese Journal of Psychosomatic Medicine, 73,* 302–311.

Hospice Foundation of America. (2018). *What is hospice?* https://hospicefoundation.org/Hospice-Care/Hospice-Services

Hunter, E. G. (2008a). Beyond death: Inheriting the past and giving to the future, transmitting the legacy of one's self. *Omega: Journal of Death and Dying, 56,* 313–329. https://doi.org/10.2190/om.56.4.a

Hunter, E. G. (2008b). Legacy: The occupational transmission of self through actions and artifacts. *Journal of Occupational Science, 15,* 48–54. https://doi.org/10.1080/14427591.2008.9686607

Jacques, N. D., & Hasselkus, B. R. (2004). The nature of occupation surrounding dying and death. *OTJR: Occupation, Participation and Health, 24,* 44–53. https://doi.org/10.1177/153944920402400202

Keesing, S., & Rosenwax, L. (2011). Is occupation missing from occupational therapy in palliative care? *Australian Journal of Occupational Therapy, 58,* 329–336. https://doi.org/10.1111/j.1440-1630.2011.00958.x

Kiresuk, T. J., & Sherman, R. E. (1968). Goal Attainment Scaling: A general method for evaluating comprehensive community mental health programs. *Community Mental Health Journal, 4,* 443–453. https://doi.org/10.1007/BF01530764

Kiresuk, T. J., Smith, A., & Cardillo, J. E. (2014). *Goal Attainment Scaling: Applications, theory, and measurement*. Psychology Press.

la Cour, K., Josephsson S., & Luborsky M. (2005). Creating connections to life during life-threatening illness: Creative activity experienced by elderly people and occupational therapists. *Scandinavian Journal of Occupational Therapy, 12,* 98–109. https://doi.org/10.1080/11038120510030889

la Cour, K., Nordell, K., & Josephson, S. (2009). Everyday lives of people with advanced cancer: Activity, time, location, and experience. *OTJR: Occupation, Participation and Health, 29,* 154–162. https://doi.org/10.3928%2F15394492-20090914-03

Law, M., Baptiste, S., Carswell, A., McColl, M., Polatajko, H., & Pollock, N. (2019). *Canadian Occupational Performance Measure* (5th ed., rev.) COPM, Inc.

Lyons, M., Orozovic, N., Davis, J., & Newman, J. (2002). Doing-being-becoming: Occupational experiences of persons with life-threatening illnesses. *American Journal of Occupational Therapy, 56,* 285–295. https://doi.org/10.5014/ajot.56.3.285

Marcil, W. M. (2006). The hospice nurse and occupational therapist: A marriage of expedience. *Home Health Care Management and Practice, 19*(1), 26–30. https://doi.org/10.1177/1084822306292514

Marcoux, J.-S. (2001). The 'casser maison' ritual: Constructing the self by emptying the home. *Journal of Material Culture, 6,* 213–235. https://doi.org/10.1177/135918350100600205

McKay, M. H. (2019). The role of occupational therapy in consultation with dementia care teams: An occupational adaptation-based approach. *SIS Quarterly Practice Connections, 4*(3), 22–24.

National Hospice and Palliative Care Organization. (2020). *Hospice facts and figures.* https://www.nhpco.org/hospice-facts-figures/

Noguchi, W., Ohno, T., Morita, S., Aihara, O., Tsujii, H., Shimozuma, K., & Matsushima, E. (2004). Reliability and validity of the Functional Assessment of Chronic Illness Therapy–Spiritual (FACIT–Sp) for Japanese patients with cancer. *Supportive Care in Cancer, 12,* 240–245. https://doi.org/10.1007/s00520-003-0582-1

Peoples, H., Brandt, A., Waehrens, E. E., & la Cour, K. (2017). Managing occupations in everyday life for people with advanced cancer living at home. *Scandinavian Journal of Occupational Therapy, 24,* 57–64. https://doi.org/10.1080/11038128.2016.1225815

Peoples, H., Nissen, N., Brandt, A., & la Cour, K. (2018). Belonging and quality of life as perceived by people with advanced cancer who live at home. *Journal of Occupational Science, 25,* 200–213. https:/doi.org/10.1080/14427591.2017.1384932

Pickens, N. D., & Long, T. (2016). Occupational therapy practitioners working with caregivers in adult palliative care and end-of-life care. *OT Practice, 21*(3), CE1–CE8.

Pizzi, M. (2001). The Pizzi Holistic Wellness Assessment. *Occupational Therapy in Health Care, 13,* 51–66. https://doi.org/10.1080/ J003v13n03_06

Pizzi, M. (2010). Promoting wellness in end-of-life care. In M. Scaffa, M. Reitz, & M. Pizzi (Eds.), *Occupational therapy in the promotion of health and wellness* (pp. 493–511). F. A. Davis.

Pizzi, M. A. (2015). Promoting health and well-being at the end of life through client-centered care. *Scandinavian Journal of Occupational Therapy, 22,* 442–449. https://doi.org/10.3109/11038128.2015.1025834

Pizzi, M. A., & Richards, L. G. (2017). Guest Editorial – Promoting health, well-being, and quality of life in occupational therapy: A commitment to a paradigm shift for the next 100 years. *American Journal of Occupational Therapy, 71,* 7104170010. https://doi.org/10.5014/ajot.2017.028456

Siebert, C. (2016a). Home health plans of care, intervention, and team collaboration. In K. Vance (Ed.), *Home health care: A guide for occupational therapy practice* (pp. 87–119). AOTA Press.

Siebert, C. (2016b). The occupational therapy evaluation process in home health. In K. Vance (Ed.), *Home health care: A guide for occupational therapy practice* (pp. 61–86). AOTA Press.

Siebert, C. (2016c). Sustainable outcomes in home health. In K. Vance (Ed.), *Home health care: A guide for occupational therapy practice* (pp. 119–128). AOTA Press.

UC San Diego Health. (2021). *Shortness of breath: Maximizing your energy.* https://myhealth.ucsd.edu/3,82477

Wilcock, A. (1998). Reflections on doing, being and becoming. *Canadian Journal of Occupational Therapy, 65,* 248–256.

World Federation of Occupational Therapists. (2016). *Position statement: Occupational therapy in end of life care.* https://www.wfot.org/resources/occupational-therapy-in-end-of-life-care

7

Caregivers and Occupational Therapy: A Vital Partnership

CATHERINE VERRIER PIERSOL, PHD, OTR/L, FAOTA

Learning Objectives

After completing this chapter, readers will be able to

- describe the multifaceted stressors experienced by families who provide care to people living with a chronic condition;
- discuss the important role of occupational therapy practitioners in supporting and educating family caregivers of people living with a chronic condition; and
- explain a conceptual framework that identifies the readiness of family caregivers to participate in the collaborative process and provides an intervention approach that meets family caregivers where they are.

Key Terms and Concepts

action plan
caregiver burden
caregiver readiness
collaboration
Competence–Environmental Press Model
co-occupation
family caregivers
family conflicts
flexibility
formal caregivers
informal caregivers
mediating factors
multidimensional context
Pearlin's Stress Process Model
primary stressors
psychoeducation–skill training approach
secondary stressors
social isolation

The majority of everyday care and support for people living with chronic disease is provided by "an adult family member or other individual who has a significant relationship with, and who provides a broad range of assistance to, an individual with a chronic or other health condition, disability, or functional limitation" (RAISE Family Caregivers Act of 2017, P. L. 115-119, § 2). Collectively referred to as ***family caregivers,*** they assume the responsibility for providing various levels and types of daily care and oversight, often without formal education and training. Family caregivers are unpaid for the services they provide, yet their work is extremely critical to the delivery of care within the health care system to those with chronic conditions (Alzheimer's Association, 2022; National Alliance for Caregiving & AARP, 2020). Conversely, ***formal caregivers*** are paid and are direct service providers or staff who are educated and trained to deliver services in a variety of settings, including skilled nursing and long-term-care facilities, assisted living facilities, adult day centers, and home health agencies.

This chapter focuses on unpaid family caregivers (i.e., ***informal caregivers***) and refers broadly to caregivers of people living with a chronic condition. Chapter content includes a general overview of family caregivers, the stressors experienced by family caregivers, occupational therapy intervention for family caregivers, and a model that facilitates a partnership between caregiver and practitioner.

Family Caregivers

Family involvement in the daily care management of a person living with a chronic condition is not new; however, the level of care has increased, and the tasks required are more complex. The trend toward shorter hospital stays and reduced nursing home placements has been attributed to the shift in care from formal to informal or family caregivers (Schultz et al., 2020). The home environment can often look like a hospital or nursing home setting, with family caregivers performing medical and nursing tasks, including the use of highly technical equipment, that were once only provided by trained and licensed health professionals in medical settings (Reinhard & Feinberg, 2015; Reinhard et al., 2012).

An estimated 53 million people in the United States, or approximately 21.3% of all American adults, serve as a family caregiver to an adult or child (or both; National Alliance for Caregiving & AARP, 2020). This statistic indicates that more than 1 in 5 American adults serve in the role of family caregiver. In addition, it is estimated that 3.4 million children in the United States younger than age 18 years provide care to an adult living in the home (National Alliance for Caregiving & AARP, 2020). Specifically for older adults with a chronic condition, about 17.7 million people in the United States serve as family caregivers (National Academies of Science, Engineering, and Medicine, 2016), with close to half providing care to a person living with Alzheimer's disease or related dementia (Alzheimer's Association, 2022; see Exhibit 7.1).

Family caregivers of people living with a chronic condition are typically older adults (mean age = 51.2 years) providing care for many hours per day. On average, spouses are the oldest caregivers (age 62.3 years), and White caregivers are older than African American, Hispanic, and Asian American caregivers (National Alliance for Caregiving & AARP, 2015). About 30% of family caregivers of those living with dementia are age 65 years or older, and two-thirds are women, of whom more than one-third are daughters of the care recipient (Alzheimer's Association, 2022). Most caregivers (66%) reside in the same household as the person living with dementia. Moreover, approximately one-quarter of people caring for a person living with dementia are considered "sandwich generation" caregivers; that is, they care for both an older adult, typically a parent, and a child or multiple children (Alzheimer's Association, 2022).

EXHIBIT 7.1.
FACTS ABOUT FAMILY CAREGIVERS

- Approximately 53 million adults in the United States (more than 1 in 5 Americans) serve as a family caregiver to an adult or child (or both).
- About 17.7 million people in the United States are the caregiver of an older adult with a chronic condition, with close to half providing care to a person living with dementia.
- These caregivers assume the responsibility for providing various levels and types of care, often without formal education and training.

Caregiving is a ***co-occupation*** that involves the participation of both the family member and the person living with a chronic condition (American Occupational Therapy Association, 2020). As the chronic condition progresses, the person's participation level changes, and the family member must assume greater responsibility. Multiple factors influence the complexity of caregiving, such as the health condition and living situation of the person with chronic disease, the competing responsibilities of the caregiver, and the amount of financial resources (National Alliance for Caregiving & AARP, 2020; Schulz et al., 2020). Caregivers assume a plethora of caregiving tasks that include providing assistance with self-care, mobility, and household tasks; offering emotional support; facilitating social connections; and managing medications, health maintenance, and care coordination (Table 7.1). Caregivers must serve as advocates and surrogates, hire and supervise paid caregivers, and arrange and manage in-home help. For people living with progressive, chronic cognitive decline, family caregivers must handle challenging behavioral symptoms that often lead to the decision to place the person in a nursing home. As a co-occupation, participation in the occupation of caregiving becomes greater for the family caregiver over the continuum of the chronic condition, causing increased stress and deterioration in well-being (Dunkle et al., 2014); thus, occupational therapy practitioners must understand and appreciate the nature of co-occupation and the need over time to provide the most effective and timely intervention.

These caregiving responsibilities demand continuous decision making, problem solving, and communication with other family members and health providers, along with attentiveness to the well-being of the person living with the chronic condition (Schulz et al., 2020). The ability to manage day-to-day tasks depends on caregiver knowledge and skills, personal health status, cultural beliefs and values, and the quality of the relationship between the caregiver and the person living with chronic disease. Because people with chronic conditions desire to remain at home and rely on unpaid support and assistance, family caregivers play a critical role in sustaining the health and well-being of those for whom they care (National Alliance for Caregiving & AARP, 2020; see Case Example 7.1). Thus, caregiving responsibilities place substantial stress, burden, and demand on the caregiver.

TABLE 7.1. Caregiver Roles and Common Associated Occupations

Caregiver Roles	Common Associated Occupations
Direct care provider	• Provides medical symptom management (e.g., dispensing medication, monitoring body and medical device systems) • Assists with ADLs (e.g., bathing, dressing, toileting, grooming, eating, shaving, bowel–bladder management, sexuality) • Helps with IADLs (e.g., cooking, shopping, running errands, completing household tasks, cleaning, reorganizing home environment)
Emotional support provider	• Provides companionship • Encourages patient self-efficacy • Includes spiritual support
Care coordinator	• Manages care across settings and providers • Schedules appointments • Provides transportation • Helps make medical decisions • Facilitates patient's understanding of care • Manages medical emergencies
Advocate	• Receives important information • Facilitates provider understanding • Helps maintain social relationships • Facilitates patient's self-care tasks
Financial manager	• Handles finances and financial issues • Helps facilitate legal support and advance care directives • Gathers resources and support

Sources. Adapted from O'Sullivan (2015) and Williams (2020). Used with permission from the American Occupational Therapy Association.
Note. ADLs = activities of daily living; IADLs = instrumental activities of daily living.

CASE EXAMPLE 7.1. DARRELL: CAREGIVER DURING END-OF-LIFE CARE

Darrell was age 52 years and the husband of **Tameka,** who was age 48 years and had liver cell carcinoma with metastases to her lungs, multiple levels of her spine, and her right hip bone. She was told during her most recent hospital stay that she was a candidate for hospice care and would likely need assistance with symptom management. Tameka chose to discharge home with hospice care.

Darrell did not know how he felt about Tameka dying at home because their young adult twin sons were living with them while attending their first year of college. However, dying at home was Tameka's stated preference, and he wanted to honor her wishes. Tameka said she wanted to make a series of videos for her two sons, as a legacy for when they get married and start their own families. Darrell worried whether she would be able to do this because he reported she was exhausted after just getting up to go to the bathroom.

Occupational therapy interventions used to help support Darrell included environmental modification strategies and durable medical equipment (DME) recommendations. Although hospice assisted with getting the DME Tameka needed, the occupational therapy practitioner reviewed with Darrell recommendations for how to modify their home environment to make best use of the DME.

Tameka preferred to be upstairs in her room to sleep, and the only bath with a walk-in shower was upstairs, in Tameka's preferred bathroom. She was able to go up and down stairs safely, despite a limp. In the recommendations for environmental modification, the occupational therapy practitioner emphasized the importance of having areas both upstairs and downstairs in which Tameka could rest in a position that minimized her pain and suggested areas where Darrell and her sons could be physically close to Tameka. Energy conservation and fatigue management education and training was provided for Darrell to help Tameka reserve the energy to complete her legacy work, help get her legal affairs in order, and spend quality time with her sons. Strategies on adapting and simplifying legacy work were also included because of the extensive project Tameka had chosen.

Education on adapting to a new normal in which new routines may be adopted in place of previous familiar routines was provided for Darrell after Tameka said she was not looking forward to continuing their morning routine of having breakfast and going for a walk; Tameka reported she did not want to be seen by their neighbors and that eggs currently made her nauseated. Instead, Tameka would drink a protein shake and walk with Darrell in their backyard.

Source. From "Caregiving," by T. Williams, in B. Braveman and R. Newman (Eds.), *Cancer and Occupational Therapy: Enabling Performance and Participation Across the Lifespan* (p. 371), 2020, AOTA Press.

STRESSORS EXPERIENCED BY FAMILY CAREGIVERS

The impact of caregiving on the family caregiver is far reaching and distinct to the person. Some caregivers report a sense of satisfaction or benefit from the care they provide that fosters expertise and confidence and promotes a positive relationship with the person receiving care (Schulz et al., 2020). Although it is important to acknowledge that caregiving can be a positive experience, much more evidence has shown the negative impact of caregiving and the burden it places on the caregiver. ***Caregiver burden*** is described as the potential negative effects that providing care can have on a caregiver's "health, emotional status, and quality of life, which often also adversely affects occupational, social, and personal roles" (Williams, 2020, p. 363).

To understand the effect that caregiving has on the family caregiver, the Chronic Disease Care Trajectory (Schulz et al., 2020), adapted from the work of Schulz and Tompkins (2010), explains the relationship between caregiver tasks and caregiver health and well-being across a continuum from sporadic care (i.e., periodic care when needed) through end-of-life care and death. As the condition progresses, the care tasks increase in number, complexity, and time and require specialty knowledge and skills, with a greater effect on caregiver stress and emotional burden. End-of-life care may include placement in a long-term-care facility. At this stage of the trajectory, caregiving tasks may include advocating for quality care, providing some personal care, and offering emotional support. Although the caregiver role is changed, family caregivers have continued burden and stress.

Caregiving can affect a person's physical and emotional health, social relationships and engagement, and employment and financial security (Schulz et al., 2020). Caregiver stress has long been reported and studied (Pearlin et al., 1981, 1990; Quayhagen & Quayhagen, 1988). ***Pearlin's Stress Process Model*** (Pearlin et al., 1990) views stress as a consequence of a process that exposes caregivers to ***primary stressors*** (i.e., those directly related to caregiving, such as managing medications) and ***secondary stressors*** (i.e., those external to the caregiver role, such as work responsibilities and personal characteristics like self-esteem and confidence) and posits that there are ***mediating factors*** (i.e., coping strategies, social supports) that support and intervene to reduce stress and promote caregiver well-being. On the basis of this model, for example, occupational therapy interventions that promote caregiver use of coping and support strategies can mediate stress and thus promote better quality of life. This conceptual framework closely aligns with the principles of and practice approaches used in palliative care.

Because of increasing stress and lack of support, ***social isolation*** is often an outcome of rising care demands. Caregivers become consumed by the responsibilities of caregiving and by default isolate themselves from family and friends. In addition, the quality of the relationship between the caregiver and the person for whom they are caring may be compromised. Particularly among spousal caregivers of persons living with dementia who exhibit behavioral symptoms such as aggression or inhibition, relationships as well as emotional and physical intimacy are affected (Ascher et al., 2010).

Social relationships are also compromised when family members have different viewpoints about the condition of and experiences with the person living with chronic disease. As such, ***family conflicts*** span a spectrum of issues that include differences of opinion about diagnosis and condition severity, disagreements about when and where to transition from home to a care facility, approaches to providing care, and lack of appreciation from other family members for the care provided (National Academies of Science, Engineering, and Medicine, 2016). External factors also affect the caregiver role and include financial resources, accessibility of services, quality of services, and available resources (National Academies of Science, Engineering, and Medicine, 2016).

Finally, the demands placed on family caregivers who are in the workforce are rising. Their impact on career aspirations primarily affects middle-aged women, who are often juggling primary caregiver responsibilities and their career goals (National Alliance for Caregiving & AARP, 2020; Schulz et al., 2020). Evidence indicates that the quality of work performance, potential for career advancement, available paid weekly work hours, and opportunity for wage increases are affected (Schulz et al., 2020). Risk factors that may affect caregiver well-being are listed in Exhibit 7.2.

Occupational Therapy Intervention for Family Caregivers

Effective caregiver interventions have been found to possess the following characteristics (Harding et al., 2011; Rouch et al., 2021; Walter & Pinquart,

EXHIBIT 7.2.
RISK FACTORS AFFECTING CAREGIVER WELL-BEING

Age

- Younger caregivers often need to balance employment with the caregiver and other roles.
- Younger caregivers and caregivers of younger patients report higher levels of interaction problems and unmet needs (Lund et al., 2015).
- Elderly caregivers report depression, poorer self-rated health, and difficulty sustaining care at home.

Gender

- Women exhibit higher levels of burden and are at greater risk for depression, anxiety, and drug use than men.
- Men often treat caregiving as a job in which they can achieve mastery, compared with women, who focus on providing physical assistance and on relationship changes.

Personality

- Caregivers who worry more than others tend to show increased distress levels.
- Extroverted caregivers may recruit more support and maintain pleasurable activities.
- Conscientious caregivers report lower levels of depression.
- Organized caregivers report lower levels of stress.

Relationship dynamics

- Preexisting relationship difficulties with the care recipient place caregivers at risk for distress.
- Spousal caregivers may have more distress if the role is expected of them than if it is freely chosen.

Caregiver health and mental status

- Older caregivers experiencing cognitive impairment often struggle with depression and difficulty sustaining care at home.
- Older caregivers are at risk for engaging in potentially harmful behaviors toward care recipients.
- Caregivers report that providing psychosocial support is stressful but that caring for a person with communication difficulties is the most stressful.

(Continued)

EXHIBIT 7.2.
RISK FACTORS AFFECTING CAREGIVER WELL-BEING *(Cont.)*

Level of care required

- An increased risk of mortality and institutionalization is associated with care recipients who need a large amount of physical, cognitive, or behavioral support over a long period of time.
- Caregivers who assist with care recipients' ADLs often demonstrate poor preventive health behaviors and decreased participation in leisure activity.
- As the level of care increases, caregiver levels of depression, general forgetfulness, excessive worry, and feelings of inadequacy often increase.

Access to resources and respite

- Caregivers confined to their home can experience decreased well-being because of physical isolation and decreased social relationships.

Stress triggers for harmful behaviors

- Higher levels of physical care over longer periods of time, cognitive impairments related to the care recipient's condition, inadequate access to community resources, and caregiver decline are associated with triggering caregiver depression, anxiety, low self-esteem, and substance abuse.
- Stress triggers place caregivers at risk for exhibiting physically or psychologically harmful behaviors, such as yelling, withholding food, threatening institutionalization, insulting, and rough handling.
- Harmful behaviors are precursors to neglect and abuse.

Note. ADLs = activities of daily living.
Source. From "Caregiving," by T. Williams, in B. Braveman and R. Newman (Eds.), *Cancer and Occupational Therapy: Enabling Performance and Participation Across the Lifespan* (p. 364), 2020, AOTA Press. Copyright © 2020 by the American Occupational Therapy Association. Adapted with permission.

2020; Zarit & Femia, 2017): a ***psychoeducation–skill training approach,*** in which caregivers actively apply and practice new knowledge and skills, receive feedback, and strategize ways to apply skills in future situations; ***multidimensional content,*** addressing numerous issues that might affect caregiver health and well-being; ***flexibility*** to address needs related to the individual caregiving situation; and an ***action plan*** for ongoing needs and strategies to address new situations as they develop (see Exhibit 7.3).

Occupational therapy intervention for family caregivers reflects these characteristics, including caregiver education, training, and advocacy and a distinct approach that helps caregivers understand the disease process, modify activities to optimize performance, and manage daily care responsibilities. Foundational to the provision of occupational therapy intervention with family caregivers is a positive therapeutic relationship, which is grounded in a collaborative approach. ***Collaboration*** is a partnership in which the practitioner and family caregiver share care planning and decision making (Haesler et al., 2010), which is also an important tenet of palliative care. In this approach, the caregiver (layperson) and the occupational therapy practitioner (professional) work as partners, learning from each other throughout the process. Through this partnership, the caregiver is empowered to assume caregiving tasks, implement care strategies, and make critical decisions.

The ***Competence–Environmental Press Model*** (Lawton & Nahemow, 1973) and its expansion in occupational therapy to include occupation (Person–Environment–Occupation Model; Law et al., 1996) provide a structure from which to approach collaboration with caregivers. The model's conceptual underpinnings are built on the tenet that characteristics of the physical environment and tasks affect people's functional competence, both positively and negatively. The model suggests that the interchange between the declining competency of the person living with

EXHIBIT 7.3.
CHARACTERISTICS OF CAREGIVER INTERVENTIONS

- *Psychoeducation–skill training approach:* Caregivers actively apply and practice new knowledge and skills, receive feedback, and strategize ways to apply skills in future situations.
- *Multidimensional content:* Addresses numerous issues that might affect caregiver health and well-being.
- *Flexibility:* Addresses individual needs related to the caregiving situation.
- *Action plan:* Addresses ongoing needs and new caregiving situations as they develop.

the chronic condition (e.g., performance skills, physical mobility, cognitive level) and the press or impact of the environment (e.g., physical barriers, clutter, low lighting) can lead to occupational dysfunction. The model posits that as a person's physical and cognitive functions decline, the press of the environment becomes greater. Thus, implementing strategies that reduce environmental press (e.g., removing clutter, using visual cues, installing adaptive equipment) can promote greater competency or occupational performance in the person living with a chronic disease. With dementia, the press of the environment can trigger behavioral symptoms that are common in people living with dementia (e.g., a bathroom that is cold in temperature and uninviting triggers agitation and refusal to take a bath). By implementing strategies that address the environmental press (e.g., warming the bathroom in advance and playing calming music during bath time), behavioral symptoms can be minimized or eliminated.

Guided by the transaction between personal competence and environmental press and applying the activity analysis process, occupational therapy practitioners are also equipped to teach caregivers strategies that promote a "just-right" fit between the capacities of the person living with a chronic condition and the demands of the activity. Among the health care interprofessional team, occupational therapy practitioners are distinguished by their expertise in analyzing the features of an activity (e.g., number of steps, required performance skills) and adapting or simplifying the demands to meet the patient's capacity. In addition to the environmental strategies discussed previously, occupational therapy practitioners can identify strategies that address optimal ways of communicating (e.g., verbal cues, visual cues, demonstration) and setting up an activity (reduce the number of steps, use a checklist) to promote successful daily care management.

It is important to teach caregivers how to modify these strategies and create new strategies as the person's chronic condition progresses; for example, as new symptoms emerge, dependency increases, or the person's condition declines overall. As the disease progresses, the initial strategies may become less effective, and new care challenges will emerge. Occupational therapy practitioners can help caregivers identify methods for recalibrating their appraisal of the situation and their capacity to be effective. One such method is the process of problem-solving. When care challenges arise, teaching caregivers to use a problem-solving approach strengthens their self-efficacy, minimizes anxiety associated with caregiving (Gitlin, 2009; Piersol et al., 2017), and offers them a skill to use when new situations occur after the occupational therapy intervention is complete.

Figure 7.1 provides a six-stage process for problem solving that begins with a description of the situation (e.g., a caregiver's mother has chronic pulmonary disease and arthritis and is no longer able to perform self-care activities independently and safely). Step 2 involves identifying the *activator,* which is the cause or multiple causes of the situation (e.g., the mother has a high level of pain in both hips and becomes easily short of breath, which is limiting her ability to complete all the steps of the morning routine). Step 3 targets the consequences of the situation (e.g., the mother becomes frustrated with her declining function and burden on her daughter, and the daughter is typically late to work because she has to spend more time helping her mother). Step 4 requires the occupational therapy practitioner and caregiver to brainstorm together and identify potential strategies (e.g., set up an environment for the mother to sit and get dressed where clothes are easily accessible, introduce the use of long-handled devices). This is where partnership is vitally important. What ideas does the caregiver bring to the problem? The caregiver's beliefs, values, and routines must be considered and should take precedence. Once strategies have been identified, Steps 5 and 6 involve trying the strategies, evaluating whether they work and revising them if necessary. Exhibit 7.4 lists common occupational therapy interventions that can support caregivers.

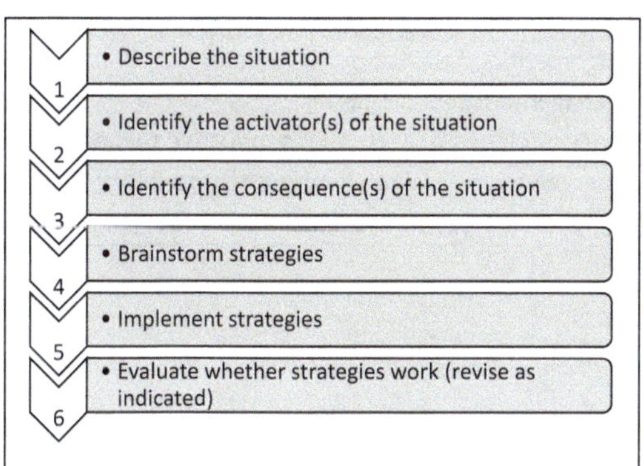

Figure 7.1 The problem-solving process with caregivers.

EXHIBIT 7.4.

OCCUPATIONAL THERAPY INTERVENTIONS THAT ARE SUPPORTIVE OF CAREGIVERS IN SPECIFIC SETTINGS

Clinic-based interventions

- Education and training on assisting with ADL, mobility, and communication needs of care recipient
- Emphasis on physical and cognitive impairment remediation and compensatory strategy training for care recipient
- Emphasis on dressing and bowel–bladder management to ease caregiver burden
- Emphasis on safety training
- Beginning behavior management training
- Beginning medication management training
- Beginning stress management and relaxation techniques
- Referral to other services, such as counseling and nutrition

Palliative care in the home

- Role balance education for caregivers; emphasis on work balance with younger caregivers and on balancing the caregiver role with other family roles
- Ability and frequency of engagement in desired and leisure activities
- Emphasis on medication management
- Development of efficient daily routines with simplification strategies
- Emphasis on addressing the need for environmental modifications and safety training
- Time management and organization training for coordinating follow-up medical care, transportation needs, and other role demands
- Stress management and relaxation techniques
- Behavior management techniques
- Skills training on telehealth and other supportive technology assistance
- Energy conservation and fatigue management training
- Emphasis on addressing community accessibility

(Continued)

EXHIBIT 7.4.
OCCUPATIONAL THERAPY INTERVENTIONS THAT ARE SUPPORTIVE OF CAREGIVERS IN SPECIFIC SETTINGS *(Cont.)*

- Skills training to access community resources and to recruit support and respite care
- Referrals to other services, such as counseling, financial, and legal management

Note. ADL = activities of daily living.
Source. Adapted from "Supporting Caregiver Identity," by T. Williams, 2016, *OT Practice, 21*(19), p. CE5.

Drawing from research describing the effectiveness of occupational therapy interventions for caregivers of people with chronic conditions (Rouch et al., 2021), depression, burden or strain, quality of life, and knowledge were the outcomes most frequently measured. Psychoeducation interventions (e.g., problem solving, coaching, case management) showed a reduction in caregiver depression and burden and an improvement in quality of life (QoL). Interventions that combined education on the disease process with skills training resulted in an improvement in caregiver QoL and knowledge and a reduction in burden. Similarly, evidence supporting occupational therapy caregiver interventions in dementia care showed an improvement in caregiver knowledge, a reduction in caregiver stress and upset, a reduction in functional dependency in the person living with dementia, and an improvement in QoL for the caregiver and person living with dementia (Piersol et al., 2017).

Framework for Implementing a Collaborative Approach With Caregivers

To effectively engage with caregivers, occupational therapy practitioners must consider the caregiver's level of readiness to participate in the therapeutic process and to assume caregiving responsibilities. ***Caregiver readiness*** is a term borrowed from the Transtheoretical Model of Behavioral

Change (Prochaska et al., 1992; Prochaska & Velicer, 1997), which explains behavior change in stages that reflect the person's readiness or intention to change what they do. The model postulates that behavior change does not occur until the person is ready and that changing behavior is complex and necessitates incremental cognitive and behavioral actions that occur at different levels of readiness. The five stages of change are as follows: (1) *precontemplation* (the person does not acknowledge that there is a problem), (2) *contemplation* (the person acknowledges that there is a problem but is not yet ready to make a change), (3) *preparation* (the person is getting ready to change behavior), (4) *action* (the person is ready to change behavior), and (5) *maintenance* (the person maintains the behavior change).

The caregiver's level of readiness to learn and implement care approaches informs and guides the collaborative approach. Caregivers at a high readiness level are immediately receptive to learning and implementing strategies, whereas those at a low readiness level first need education to understand the condition and are not yet ready to learn new skills. To be an effective partner, occupational therapy practitioners must avoid the pitfall of judging a caregiver's behavior as "lacking motivation," "not following through with recommendations," or "disinterested"; rather the practitioner needs to step back, reflect, and identify the caregiver's level of readiness and meet them there.

Educating and working with caregivers requires that caregivers practice and implement new, potentially unfamiliar care techniques to manage the chronic condition, including medications, medical appointments, and daily care management. Drawing on the stages of change offers occupational therapy practitioners a mechanism for meeting caregivers where they are—that is, a way to approach the caregiver and provide intervention that will be accepted and facilitate a change in readiness. Family caregivers can enter the therapeutic process at any stage of readiness. Figure 7.2 identifies each caregiver readiness level and the suggested therapeutic approach.

Understanding the level of caregiver readiness initially informs the approach to instructing the caregiver about the condition and the use of strategies. Caregivers at a preparation stage are ready and receptive to learn and implement strategies, whereas caregivers at a precontemplative level need education to understand the condition and are not ready to learn new skills. For example, a caregiver with a low level of readiness

CAREGIVER READINESS LEVEL		APPROACH WITH CAREGIVER
1. **Precontemplation** • Lacks knowledge about the condition • Feels everything is fine • Not sure about being caregiver	Not ready	• Start with basic education about condition • Identify needs for learning • Discuss what would make the situation better
2. **Contemplation** • Aware problem exists but lack knowledge about the disease • Trying to understand and thinking about taking action	Unsure	• Identify immediate concern • Introduce basic information about the condition • Introduce simple care approaches, e.g., establish a daily routine
3. **Preparation** • Intending to take action • Asking questions about disease and how to manage daily routine	Ready	• Provide information about the condition • Problem-solve potential approaches • Practice and refine care approaches
4. **Action &** 5. **Maintenance** • Active participation • Modifies behavior and environment • Generalizes strategies to another problem	Take action and sustain	• Validate actions; explain what works and why • Prepare for future care challenges as condition progresses

Figure 7.2 Caregiver readiness and therapeutic approach.

may need more education about the chronic disease and its symptoms. A caregiver at a low level of readiness may need more time before introducing specific strategies such as modifying the home environment or changing the way they communicate with their family member. Caregivers at a high level of readiness tend to be immediately receptive to strategies and to come up with their own ideas. Often these types of caregivers are labeled as "doing well . . . doesn't really need intervention." In reality, caregivers at this high level do benefit from validation of what they are doing—and often the opportunity to understand why the strategy they are using is working. In dementia care, family caregivers who are knowledgeable about dementia and exhibit readiness to try new strategies will benefit from different types of education and training than those with little knowledge of dementia or limited readiness to change.

Gitlin and Rose (2016) explored factors associated with the level of readiness of caregivers of people living with dementia. Caregivers at a high level of readiness had better mood and less financial difficulty, which were associated with the person living with dementia having lower cognitive ability and more behavioral symptoms. This study also showed that therapeutic engagement and perceived benefits of the intervention enhanced the probability of change in caregiver readiness. This finding supports the importance of approaching family caregivers as partners and using a collaborative approach with all caregivers of people living with a chronic condition. Regardless of the condition, occupational therapy practitioners must consider the caregiver's level of readiness and meet the caregiver where they are while fostering their transition through the stages of change (Gitlin & Rose, 2016).

Summary

The majority of everyday care and support for people living with chronic disease is provided by family caregivers who are unpaid and typically do not have the knowledge and skills to provide the necessary care. Often the home environment of the person living with a chronic condition slowly transitions to look more like a medical setting than a home, with families performing tasks that were once provided by health care professionals. Occupational therapy practitioners can play an important role in educating, training, and supporting family caregivers as they assume the plethora of caregiving responsibilities, from personal care to managing medical appointments. Case Example 7.2 describes Marla, who is caring for her mother, Mrs. Soto. Marla has gradually assumed more and more responsibilities over the past 4 years, since Mrs. Soto moved into her home. The case example highlights key aspects of palliative care services and the collaborative approach of the occupational therapist, who meets Marla where she is to build her caregiving skills and confidence.

CASE EXAMPLE 7.2. MARLA: CAREGIVER TO AN OLDER ADULT WITH DEMENTIA

Marla is caring for her 81-year-old mother, **Mrs. Soto.** Marla is age 53 years, is divorced, and shares custody of her two adolescent children. She has been a high school teacher at the local high school for almost 30 years. Mrs. Soto was diagnosed with vascular dementia 6 years ago, although Marla started noticing changes in her mother's memory before the diagnosis. Mrs. Soto's dementia is in the middle to late stage. She also has chronic osteoarthritis that causes significant pain in her hips and knees when she is being washed and dressed.

(Continued)

CASE EXAMPLE 7.2. MARLA: CAREGIVER TO AN OLDER ADULT WITH DEMENTIA *(Cont.)*

Mrs. Soto moved into Marla's home almost 4 years ago. Her bedroom and bathroom are on the second floor. After 6 months of living with Marla, Mrs. Soto began to attend an Adult Day Center (ADC) 3 days a week. When she could no longer be at home alone, she started attending the day program Monday through Friday. She enjoyed the center for almost 3 years; most recently, though, the staff recommended Mrs. Soto be placed on palliative care at home. At first, Marla was a bit hesitant to agree with this plan; however, after learning more about palliative care and speaking at length with the ADC director and her mother's physician, she agreed that this transition was the best for her mother. Marla was fortunate to be able to take a 3-month leave of absence from work to settle her mom at home and collaborate with the palliative care team.

Palliative care services were initiated at home and included occupational therapy. Using a collaborative approach, the occupational therapist established rapport and laid the foundation for shared care planning and decision making. The occupational therapist visited Mrs. Soto and Marla to complete the evaluation and identify the care plan with Marla. She spent time talking with Marla to understand her experiences and identify her current caregiving concerns. Marla had some knowledge of dementia and asked appropriate questions to learn more. She demonstrated a readiness to engage in the therapeutic process and implement caregiving strategies. After the home visit, reflecting on her interactions and observations, the occupational therapist rated Marla's readiness as 3–preparatory stage.

The occupational therapy intervention plan focused on promoting quality of life for both Marla and Mrs. Soto. The immediate need expressed by Marla was to move her mother to the first floor so her mother would not need to go to the second floor, and she would not need to go up and down the stairs. The occupational therapist worked with Marla to plan and implement modifications to the environment and to identify adaptive equipment and other equipment needs. During this process, Marla became a bit overwhelmed; in response, the occupational therapist stepped back and moved at a slower pace, reinforcing the rationale for the first-floor set-up and adjusting the plan through discussion with Marla. Once the change was made, Marla was happy and realized how much more efficient the new set-up was for her and the paid caregiver.

Other areas that were addressed in occupational therapy were Mrs. Soto's increase in sleep and lack of activity. Marla was frustrated that her mother was

(Continued)

CASE EXAMPLE 7.2. MARLA: CAREGIVER TO AN OLDER ADULT WITH DEMENTIA *(Cont.)*

sleeping most of the day, as reported by the paid caregiver. She knew sleeping tended to increase as the disease progressed, but she talked to the occupational therapist and expressed her concern about her mother's sleeping more during the day. The occupational therapist used the problem-solving process with Marla to explore why her mother was sleeping more, which revealed there was no specific routine during the day, and activities were too complicated for Mrs. Soto to perform. Together, Marla and the occupational therapist generated strategies that established a daily activity routine (including naps) and reduced the complexity of the activities so Mrs. Soto was able to engage. Marla was able to practice strategies and get feedback from the occupational therapist, which increased her skills. Included in the strategies were physical cueing and positioning strategies that minimized Mrs. Soto's experience of pain.

While working with the occupational therapist, Marla shared that her mother had started displaying mild agitation during self-care activities. Reinforcing the use of problem solving, the occupational therapist worked with Marla to identify potential causes of the agitation (e.g., rushing through the self-care activity, experiencing arthritic pain when moving, initiating morning self-care at different times each day, disorganization of the room). The occupational therapist provided education about the effect of dementia on activity performance, the benefit of a consistent daily routine, and how environmental press (e.g., clutter, disorganization) could influence her mother's agitation. In collaboration, they identified and practiced strategies to reduce the potential for Mrs. Soto to become agitated, such as establishing a set self-care morning routine that is performed the same way each morning, starting the morning routine earlier to minimize the need to rush, and organizing supplies and equipment in the room to facilitate ease of performance.

In summary, the occupational therapist used a collaborative approach to promote skill building and confidence, reduce burden and stress, and improve quality of life. The palliative care intervention focused on promoting quality of life for both Marla and Mrs. Soto through collaboration and validation of Marla's knowledge and actions. The occupational therapist initially identified Marla's high readiness (3–preparatory stage) to engage and implement care strategies. As the collaboration continued, she adjusted her approach to meet Marla where she was in terms of knowledge, skills, and perceived burden. The occupational therapy intervention resulted in improved quality of life for Marla and her mother, improved caregiver knowledge and skills, and reduced caregiver burden.

Catherine Verrier Piersol, PhD, OTR/L, FAOTA, is Professor and Chair in the Department of Occupational Therapy, Jefferson College of Rehabilitation Sciences at Thomas Jefferson University in Philadelphia, Pennsylvania.

REFERENCES

Alzheimer's Association. (2022). 2022 *Alzheimer's disease facts and figures*. https://www.alz.org/media/Documents/alzheimers-facts-and-figures.pdf

American Occupational Therapy Association. (2020). Occupational therapy practice framework: Domain and process (4th ed.). *American Journal of Occupational Therapy, 74*(Suppl. 2), 7412410010. https://doi.org/10.5014/ajot.2020.74S2001

Ascher, E. A., Sturm, V. E., Seider, B. H., Holley, S. R., Miller, B. L., & Levenson, R. W. (2010). Relationship satisfaction and emotional language in frontotemporal dementia and Alzheimer disease patients and spousal caregivers. *Alzheimer Disease and Associated Disorders, 24,* 49–55. https://doi.org/10.1097/WAD.0b013e3181bd66a3

Dunkle, R. E., Feld, S., Lehning, A. J., Kim, H., Shen, H. W., & Kim, M. H. (2014). Does becoming an ADL spousal caregiver increase the caregiver's depressive symptoms? *Research on Aging, 36,* 655–682. https://doi.org/10.1177/0164027513516152

Gitlin, L. (2009). Problem solving: A teaching and therapeutic tool for older adults and their families. In J. Söderback (Ed.), *Handbook of occupational therapy interventions* (pp. 415–429). Springer Science.

Gitlin, L. N., & Rose, K. (2016). Impact of caregiver readiness on outcomes of a nonpharmacological intervention to address behavioral symptoms in persons with dementia. *International Journal of Geriatric Psychiatry, 31,* 1056–1063. https://doi.org/10.1002/gps.4422

Haesler, E., Bauer, M., & Nay, R. (2010). Recent evidence on the development and maintenance of constructive staff–family relationships in the care of older people—A report on a systematic review update. *International Journal of Evidence-Based Healthcare, 8,* 45–74. https://www.ncbi.nlm.nih.gov/books/NBK79951/

Harding, R., List, S., Epiphaniou, E., & Jones, H. (2011). How can informal caregivers of cancer and palliative care be supported? An updated systematic literature review of interventions and their effectiveness. *Palliative Medicine, 26,* 7–22. https://doi.org/10.1177/0269216311409613

Law, M., Cooper, B., Strong, S., Stewart, D., Rigby, P., & Letts, L. (1996). The Person–Environment–Occupation Model: A transactive approach to occupational performance. *Canadian Journal of Occupational Therapy, 63,* 9–23. https://doi.org/10.1177/000841749606300103

Lawton, M. P., & Nahemow, L. E. (1973). Ecology and the aging process. In C. Eisdorfer & M. P. Lawton (Eds.), *The psychology of adult development and aging* (pp. 619–674). American Psychological Association. https://doi.org/10.1037/10044-020

Lund, L., Ross, L., Peterson, M. A., & Groenvold, M. (2015). The interaction between informal cancer caregivers and health care professionals: A survey of caregivers' experiences of problems and unmet needs. *Support Cancer Care, 23,* 1719–1733. https://doi.org/10.1007/s00520-014-2529-0

National Academies of Sciences, Engineering, and Medicine. (2016). *Families caring for an aging America.* National Academies Press. https://doi.org/10.17226/23606

National Alliance for Caregiving & AARP. (2020). *Caregiving in the U.S.* https://www.aarp.org/content/dam/aarp/ppi/2020/05/full-report-caregiving-in-the-united-states.doi.10.26419-2Fppi.00103.001.pdf

O'Sullivan, A. (2015). Collaborating with family caregivers in the home setting. *OT Practice, 20*(11), CE1–CE7.

Pearlin, L. I., Menaghan, E. G., Lieberman, M. A., & Mullan, J. T. (1981). The stress process. *Journal of Health and Social Behavior, 22,* 337–356. https://doi.org/10.2307/2136676

Pearlin, L. I., Mullan, J. T., Semple, S. J., & Skaff, M. M. (1990). Caregiving and the stress process: An overview of concepts and their measures. *The Gerontologist, 30,* 583–594. https://doi.org/10.1093/geront/30.5.583

Piersol, C. V., Connor, S., Giller, I., Kanton, K., Lipman, S., & Seager, S. (2017). Effectiveness of interventions for caregivers of people with Alzheimer's disease and related major neurocognitive disorders: A systematic review. *American Journal of Occupational Therapy, 71,* 7105180020. https://doi.org/10.5014/ajot.2017.027581

Prochaska, J. O., DiClemente, C. C., & Norcross, J. C. (1992). In search of how people change: Applications to addictive behaviors. *American Psychologist, 47*(9), 1102–1114. https://doi.org/10.1037/0003-066X.47.9.1102

Prochaska, J. O., & Velicer, W. F. (1997). The Transtheoretical Model of health behavior change. *American Journal of Health Promotion, 12,* 38–48. https://doi.org/10.4278/0890-1171-12.1.38

Quayhagen, M. P., & Quayhagen, M. (1988). Alzheimer's stress: Coping with the caregiving role. *The Gerontologist, 28,* 391–396. https://doi.org/10.1093/geront/28.3.391

RAISE Family Caregivers Act, Pub. L. 115-119, 132 Stat. 23. (2017).

Reinhard, S. C., & Feinberg, L. (2015). The escalating complexity of family caregiving: Meeting the challenge. In J. E. Gaugler & R. L. Kane (Eds.), *Family caregiving in the new normal* (pp. 291–304). Academic Press.

Reinhard, S. C., Levine, C., & Samis, S. (2012). *Home alone: Family caregivers providing complex chronic care*. United Hospital Fund. https://uhfnyc.org/publications/publication/home-alone-family-caregivers-providing-complex-chronic-care/

Rouch, S. A., Fields, B. E., Alibrahim, H. A., Rodakowski, J., & Leland, N. E. (2021). Evidence for the effectiveness of interventions for caregivers of people with chronic conditions: A systematic review. *American Journal of Occupational Therapy, 75*, 7504190030. https://doi.org/10.5014/ajot.2021.042838

Schulz, R., Beach, S. R., Czaja, S. J., Martire, L. M., & Monin, J. K. (2020). Family caregiving for older adults. *Annual Review of Psychology, 71*, 635–659. https://doi.org/10.1146/annurev-psych-010419-050754

Schulz, R., & Tompkins, C. A. (2010). Informal caregivers in the United States: Prevalence, caregiver characteristics, and ability to provide care. In *The role of human factors in home health care: Workshop summary* (pp. 117–143). National Academies Press. https://www.ncbi.nlm.nih.gov/books/NBK210048/

Walter, E., & Pinquart, M. (2020). How effective are dementia caregiver interventions? An updated comprehensive meta-analysis. *The Gerontologist, 60*, e609–e619. https://doi.org/10.1093/geront/gnz118

Williams, T. (2016). Supporting caregiver identity. *OT Practice, 21*(19), CE1–CE8.

Williams, T. (2020). Caregiving. In B. Braveman & R. Newman (Eds.), *Cancer and occupational therapy: Enabling performance and participation across the lifespan* (pp. 361–374). AOTA Press.

Zarit, S., & Femia, E. (2017). Behavioral and psychosocial interventions for family caregivers. *Journal of Social Work Education, 44*, 49–57. https://doi.org/10.5175/JSWE.2008.773247711

Index

Note. Page numbers in *italics* indicate exhibits, figures, and tables.

I

K

L

FSC
www.fsc.org
MIX
Papier | Fördert gute Waldnutzung
FSC® C083411

Zeitfracht Medien GmbH
Ferdinand-Jühlke-Straße 7
99095 Erfurt, Deutschland
produktsicherheit@kolibri360.de